Epidemiology by Design

Epidemiology by Design

A Causal Approach to the Health Sciences

DANIEL WESTREICH

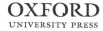
OXFORD
UNIVERSITY PRESS

Oxford University Press is a department of the University of Oxford. It furthers
the University's objective of excellence in research, scholarship, and education
by publishing worldwide. Oxford is a registered trade mark of Oxford University
Press in the UK and certain other countries.

Published in the United States of America by Oxford University Press
198 Madison Avenue, New York, NY 10016, United States of America.

CIP data is on file at the Library of Congress
ISBN 978-0-19-066576-0

Printed by Marquis, Canada

CONTENTS

ACKNOWLEDGMENTS

Professional. So, if I know anything at all about teaching, it is what I have picked up along the way from my own teachers: first and foremost I must thank them. First, those who taught me epidemiologic methods in class: Wayne Rosamond, Beverly Levine, Charlie Poole, Jane Schroeder, Jay Kaufman, Steve Marshall, William Miller, and Michele Jonsson-Funk. The textbooks I learned from (and continue to learn from) included *Epidemiology: An Introduction* by Kenneth J. Rothman; *Modern Epidemiology* (3rd edition) by Rothman, Sander Greenland, and Timothy L. Lash; and *Causal Inference* by Miguel Hernán and James Robins. I recommend reading all three books.

Next some key mentors: my doctoral advisor Annelies Van Rie (as well as the members of my doctoral committee who have not yet been mentioned: Prof. Patrick MacPhail and Joseph Eron). My postdoctoral advisor Stephen R. Cole, to this day a trusted mentor, collaborator, and friend, and who in particular I want to credit with introducing me to key ideas in causal inference and suggesting I teach risks and incidence rates from the survival curve.

Some peers in my learning process included Kim Powers, Abby Norris-Turner, Brian Pence, Elizabeth Torrone, Christy Avery, Aaron Kipp, Chanelle Howe—and too many more to name.

My frequent collaborators, including some of the above as well as Michael Hudgens, Adaora Adimora, Enrique Schisterman, Robert Platt, Elizabeth Stuart, Jessie Edwards, Alex Keil, Alex Breskin, Catherine Lesko, and some of those already named, all of whom have taught and challenged me.

At the University of North Carolina at Chapel Hill, my Chairs Andy Olshan and Til Stürmer; Nancy Colvin and Valerie Hudock; and my many faculty peers, who are a delight to work with.

My former students, who have certainly taught me more than I taught them, including Alex Breskin, Mariah Kalmin, Jordan Cates, Sabrina Zadrozny, Ruth Link-Gelles, Elizabeth T. Rogawski McQuade, Cassidy Henegar, as well as numerous others—including current students.

Noel Weiss, for helping set me on this path many years ago. Allen Wilcox, for general encouragement, and for publishing my first epidemiologic writing (a sonnet!) in a journal. Moyses Szklo, for his unending support. Jeff Martin, Martina Morris, and Steve Goodreau for their encouragement. Sandro Galea and

Katherine Keyes, for showing me it could be done. Steve Mooney, for being on this long, weird journey with me. Stanley Eisenstat, for helping teach me how to think. And anyone, at UNC and Duke and the Society for Epidemiologic Research (especially Sue Bevan and Courtney Long!) and at *American Journal of Epidemiology* and *Epidemiology* and other journals, who helped guide my way.

This book is framed within causal inference: here, I owe a particular debt of influence to what I have learned in person and from the publications of several people not already named above, including (alphabetically, and incompletely) Maria Glymour, Ashley Naimi, Judea Pearl, Maya Petersen, Sonia Hernández-Díaz, Eric Tchetgen Tchetgen, Tyler VanderWeele, as well as the Causal Inference Research Lab crew and others. My mistakes, of course, remain my own.

Finally, a big thank you to Chad Zimmerman at Oxford University Press who nurtured this project from its inception.

Peer reviewers. This book is deeply indebted to the volunteer labor of numerous epidemiologists (and occasionally others) who helped review chapters and gave selflessly of their expertise.

Round 1 peer reviewers: Charlie Poole, Stephen R. Cole, Molly Rosenberg, Jay S. Kaufman, Katherine Keyes, Matt Fox, Alex Breskin, John Jackson, Stephen Mooney, Beverly Levine, Elizabeth Torrone, Chanelle Howe, Alex Keil, Brian Pence, Holly Stewart, Ali Rowhani-Rahbar, Ghassan Hamra, Jacob Bor, Joanna Asia Maselko, Elizabeth T. Rogawski McQuade, Catherine Lesko, Jessie Edwards.

Round 2 peer reviewers: Katie Mollan, Hanna Jardel, Emma Elizabeth Navajas, Joelle Atere-Roberts, Jake Thistle. And thanks to all EPID 710 students in the Fall of 2018, who put up with a half-baked textbook. It is now, I promise you, at least two-thirds baked.

Round 3 peer reviewers: Christy Avery, Renee Heffron, Maria Mori Brooks, Rachel Ross, Alex Breskin, Sheree Schwartz, Julia Marcus, M. Maria Glymour, Stephen Mooney, Mariah Kalmin, Lynne Messer, Jordan Cates.

Personal. My dear friends and community who encouraged this work: among them Melissa Hudgens, Emily McGinty, Michael Bell Ruvinsky, Laura Wiederhoeft, Jana Hirsch, Josie Ballast, Sammy Sass, Rose Campagnola, Ethan Zoller, Cheryl Trooskin, Hilary Turnberg, Emma Kaywin, the Bozos, and many others.

My family: Dad and Dale, Mom, Luke and Anne Marie, Marilyn and Carlos, Dave and Naomi, Erica and Deron, Mary and Mario, Lily.

And my home: Katie, and Eli, and Nova. I love you.

Overview

The study of epidemiology is, to a large extent, about learning to ask good questions in population health. To do this we first must understand how to measure population health, both in a single sample (Chapter 1) and when comparing aspects of population health between two groups (Chapter 2).

This dispensed with, we consider what makes a "good question." In this work, we regard a good question, broadly, as one which is specific and well-formed, and therefore which can be answered rigorously. And one which, answered rigorously, will lead us to better population health outcomes. We mean these as guidelines, not dogmatically as rules: there are excellent questions in epidemiology and population health generally which do not meet all of these guidelines. We do, however, believe that when questions do not meet these guidelines, it is incumbent on scientists to probe the nature of the question at hand to see if it can be refined to better meet these guidelines.

In line with this, the view of this text is that most (by no means all) of the questions we want to ask in epidemiology are fundamentally causal in nature (Chapter 3), rather than predictive or descriptive (Chapter 4). But it is worth calling out that the process by which causal questions emerge often flows from description of what's happening (often in the form of public health surveillance of the world at a single time point) or prediction about what might happen: both these approaches can help us to develop causal hypotheses about how to improve health or direct us to populations in which there is the greatest need to invest resources for improved health.

How do we learn to ask better questions? "Intuition accelerators" are one name for methods which help us to think more clearly about our research questions and which help us to understand the world more fully. As an example, understanding randomized trials (Chapter 5) can help us form good research questions even when we aren't conducting a randomized trial ourselves. Specifically, it is often much easier to understand how to frame an observational data analysis (such as those discussed in Chapters 6–8) by articulating a hypothetical randomized trial that would address the question of interest. I personally find that nearly all study designs are intuition accelerators for some other aspect of epidemiologic methodology, especially around biases. This is a—if not *the*—key reason that this book is organized around study designs.

Finally, in considering what makes a good question, we should consider the ultimate impact of our scientific studies: not just in the small sample of people we are studying, but in the larger population as well, and under more realistic conditions than a small controlled study environment typically admits (Chapter 9).

A commentary by Kaufman and Hernán in the journal *Epidemiology* was titled (paraphrasing Picasso) "Epidemiologic Methods Are Useless: They Can Only Give You Answers." This book, then, hopes to teach you not just epidemiologic methods, but also—by doing so—how to ask better questions.

We now describe in slightly more detail the three sections of the text and the chapters of each section.

SECTION I: INTRODUCTION AND BACKGROUND

In this first section of the book, we lay the groundwork for understanding how study designs work, what they estimate, and how they can fail. To do so, we give an overview of prevalence and incidence, measures of contrast, causal inference, diagnostic testing, screening, and surveillance.

In Chapter 1, we describe prevalence and incidence in single samples (a single population), as well as how to quantify these measures. For incidence in particular we focus on the survival curve as the central measure of incidence of disease over time in a population and then describe how simpler measures such as the incidence proportion (i.e., the risk), incidence rate, incidence odds, and measures such as relative time can be derived from the survival curve.

In Chapter 2, we discuss measures of contrast between two groups within our population; whereas in Chapter 1 we might describe the total number of cases of disease in a large population as a whole, here we are interested in (for example) contrasting risk among those exposed to a drug and those unexposed to that drug within our large population. In this chapter, we primarily focus on difference and ratio measures. This chapter introduces the 2 × 2 table, a widely used tool for learning epidemiologic methods.

Chapter 3 discusses basic concepts in causal inference, beginning with an introduction to potential outcomes and definitions of causal contrasts (or causal estimates of effect). We discuss sufficient conditions for estimation of causal effects (which are sometimes called *causal identification conditions*), causal directed acyclic graphs (sometimes called *causal diagrams*), four key types of systematic error (confounding bias, missing data bias, selection bias, and measurement error/information bias), and we briefly discuss alternative approaches to causal inference.

Finally, in Chapter 4, we discuss concepts in diagnostic testing, screening, and disease surveillance, including concepts of sensitivity, specificity, and positive and negative predictive value. In this chapter, we briefly touch on differences between clinical epidemiology and public health epidemiology.

In Chapters 1 and 2, we assume for simplicity and conceptual clarity that all variables (including exposures, outcomes, and covariates) are measured correctly. In Chapter 3, we introduce issues related to measurement error in causal inference; in Chapter 4, we address issues of measurement in more detail. In all these chapters, and indeed in the book in general, we will be primarily concerned with dichotomous outcomes: those with two clear categories such as "alive or dead" and "diagnosed with cancer or not diagnosed with cancer." However, we will give some space to continuous outcomes—especially time to an event—in Chapters 1 and 2.

SECTION II: EPIDEMIOLOGY BY DESIGN

In the second section of the book, we build on the core concepts of measuring disease and assessing causality to describe the study designs that are the core tools of epidemiology.

In Chapter 5, we describe randomized trials. We give a broad overview of types of trials, steps in conducting a trial, and describe how trials meet (and fail to meet) core causal identification conditions. We provide a brief introduction to analysis of randomized trial data. We introduce factorial trials as well as subgroup analysis of trials as a way of explaining differences between causal interaction and effect measure modification. Finally, we describe issues in the generalizability and transportability of trials and quantitative approaches to these issues.

In Chapter 6, we address observational cohort studies in much the same way as the previous chapter addressed trials: types of cohort studies, steps in conducting such a study, the ways in which such studies meet or do not meet causal identification conditions, and a brief introduction to analysis. We expand our discussion of interaction and effect measure modification, as well as generalizability, in this setting.

In Chapter 7, we echo the structure of the previous two chapters to discuss case-control studies. Here, our focus will be on understanding the relationship between cohort studies and case-control studies and how the interpretation of the odds ratio estimated from the case-control study depends on the relationship of the case-control study to a cohort study and how controls are sampled.

Chapter 8 briefly discusses several other key study designs, including systematic reviews, meta-analysis, case-crossover, case reports and series, cross-sectional studies, and quasi-experiments.

SECTION III: FROM PATIENTS TO POLICY

Chapter 9 discusses the causal impact approach to epidemiologic methods for moving from internally valid estimates to externally valid estimates to valid estimates of the effects of population interventions. Then we briefly address the lessons of the previous chapters for the so-called hierarchy of evidence (hierarchy of study designs).

Introduction and Background

1

Measuring Disease

Epidemiology is largely concerned with the study of the presence and occurrence
of disease and ways to prevent disease and maintain health. Our first task, therefore, is to understand in some depth the concepts of prevalence and incidence,
how to quantify them, and the key types of error that can affect measurements
of each. *Prevalence* (Section 1.1) is about the presence or absence of a disease or
other factors in a population. *Incidence* (Section 1.2), on the other hand, is about
how many new cases of a disease arise over a particular time period. Both are
measurements in data, and both can be subject to various kinds of error, both *systematic error* and *random error* (Section 1.3).

Before we go into more depth on these concepts, however, it will be useful to explain the idea of a cohort—in which prevalence and incidence are typically measured.
A *cohort* is any group of people, usually followed through time; this might be a study
population in an observational or randomized study or another group of individuals.
Epidemiologists speak of both closed and open cohorts. For our purposes, a *closed
cohort* is a cohort where we start following everyone at the same time point. For example, we could start following individuals on their 40th birthdays; alternatively, we
could start following them at time of randomization in a randomized trial. Further,
a closed cohort never adds new members after enrollment ends; for example, no one
is added to the "start on your 40th birthday" cohort on their 43rd birthday. As such,
over time, a closed cohort either stays the same size or gets smaller (as people drop
out of or exit a study, or die). An *open cohort* for our purposes is one that may add
more people over time and so may get larger or smaller over time. For the remainder
of the text, if we do not specify whether we are discussing a closed or open cohort,
the reader should assume we are discussing a closed cohort.

In the remainder of the chapter, we will discuss prevalence and ways to measure
it, incidence and ways to measure it, and the broad categories of error, systematic
and random, which can affect both.

1.1 PREVALENCE

Prevalence is a description of the extent to which some factor—an exposure
or a disease condition—is present in a population. For example, we might ask
about the prevalence of obesity in a population: what we are asking about is the

Epidemiology by Design: A Causal Approach to the Health Sciences. Daniel Westreich, Oxford
University Press (2020). © Oxford University Press.
DOI: 10.1093/oso/9780190665760.001.0001

proportion or, alternately, *number of people currently living in that population who are obese.*

Broadly, prevalence is discussed as either *point prevalence* or *period prevalence.* Point prevalence is the prevalence of a disease at a single point in time, whereas period prevalence is the prevalence of a disease over a period of time. Of course, as the duration over which prevalence is considered shrinks, period prevalence will converge to point prevalence. On the other hand, point prevalence is often operationalized (put into practice) as "period prevalence over a reasonably short time window." For example, if you want to know the prevalence of HIV infection in a cohort of 1,000 people, it is difficult to imagine getting blood samples to test from all those people simultaneously (e.g., if all 1,000 participants give blood at exactly 1:00 PM this Friday). In practice, you would obtain blood samples over as short a time period as possible and test them thereafter. Alternatively, you could also define such a prevalence as "point prevalence at time of testing" while acknowledging that the testing occurred at a different calendar time for each participant.

One key circumstance when point prevalence can and should be measured is at the beginning of a research study, such as the moment after participants are enrolled in a randomized trial (Chapter 5) or observational cohort study (Chapter 6). Specifically, it is often relatively straightforward to estimate the point prevalence of a disease such as anemia at baseline (first) study visit.[1] A second circumstance when point prevalence can be measured is in a large electronic medical record database: the prevalence of a particular disease or other condition (e.g., smoking) can be assessed in all existing records in the database today—or on any other day of interest.

We measure prevalence using three main types of quantities: proportions, odds, and counts. A *prevalence proportion* is a measure of the percentage of the population that presently has the disease or who presently has a history of the disease of a specified duration in the past (e.g., "history of cancer in the past 10 years"). Since at fewest none and at most all of the members of a population can have a condition or a history of that condition, the prevalence proportion ranges from 0 to 1, much like a probability. This is the most common and perhaps clearest way of expressing prevalence, and we can assume this definition when "prevalence" is used without further explanation. It is typically what is meant by "prevalence rate," as well (see Box 1.1, well below). Prevalence proportions are sometimes expressed using simple numbers instead of percentages for ease of communication. For example, instead of reporting that 4% of the US population is living with

---

1. However, as we noted earlier, the baseline study visit will not occur at the same calendar time (or at the same age!) for all study participants; thus, such a prevalence is only a point prevalence on the timescale of the study. At the same time, it might be a period prevalence on the timescale of the calendar or age. Every observation exists on multiple timescales at once—as noted, the time of baseline study visit, day of the year, and age are all timescales operating simultaneously and are not precisely aligned with each other. You can consider how a cohort, therefore, may be considered closed on some timescales but open on others.

BOX 1.1

WHAT ARE ODDS, AND WHY?

In mathematical terms, an *odds* is defined as a function of a probability P such that odds = $P/(1 - P)$. Thus, if the probability is 5% or 0.05, then the equivalent odds is $0.05/(1 - 0.05) = 0.05/0.95 = 0.053$. If probability is 10% or 0.10, then the equivalent odds is $0.10/(1 - 0.10) = 0.1/0.9 = 0.11$. If probability is 0.25, odds is $0.25/0.75 = 0.33$ (sometimes expressed as 1:3). If probability is 0.50, then odds is $0.5/0.5 = 1$ (sometimes 1:1 or "even odds"), and a probability of 0.75 is equivalent to an odds of $0.75/0.25 = 3$ (3:1). Where probability is constrained to [0, 1], odds can range from 0 to infinity. Figure 1.1 illustrates the relationship between a probability (x-axis) and the odds (y-axis), which likewise applies to both the relationship between prevalence proportion and prevalence odds and the relationship between incidence proportion and incidence odds (see Section 1.2 for more on incidence).

You may observe that at low probability (e.g., 0.05), the odds are quite similar to the probability (0.053), but as probability increases (e.g., 0.80), the odds looks increasingly dissimilar ($0.80/0.20 = 4$). The usual guideline is that when $P \leq 0.10$ in all strata of all relevant variables (not just overall!), odds is a reasonable proxy for probability; when $P > 0.10$, more caution is needed. This is evident on the right-most panel of Figure 1.1, in which both axes are shown log-scale: this rule of thumb is shown as the (nearly) straight line between (0.01, 0.01) and (0.1, 0.1).

Why do people report odds instead of probabilities? They are convenient in gambling, of course, but the more likely reason is that they are often easier to estimate and have some convenient statistical properties. While we omit discussion of those properties here, we encourage you to seek out some of the many works on this subject to supplement this book, including Bland and Altman (2000) and Greenland (1987).

chronic obstructive pulmonary disease (COPD), we might instead report that 40 out of 1,000 Americans live with COPD.

A *prevalence odds* is a simple function of the prevalence proportion, just as the odds in general is a simple function of probability (see Box 1.2), and are typically reported out of convenience or for their desirable statistical properties. The prevalence odds, then, is simply the *prevalence proportion divided by 1 minus the prevalence proportion*. Prevalence odds will approximate the prevalence proportion when the prevalence proportion is low but may otherwise overstate prevalence proportion. As shown in Figure 1.1, as the prevalence proportion (the probability, on the x-axis) ranges from 0 to 1, the prevalence odds (y-axis) ranges from 0 to infinity (not shown, because space in this book is finite).

A *prevalence count* is exactly what it sounds like: a count of the number of cases of disease present in a population at a point in time or over a short period.

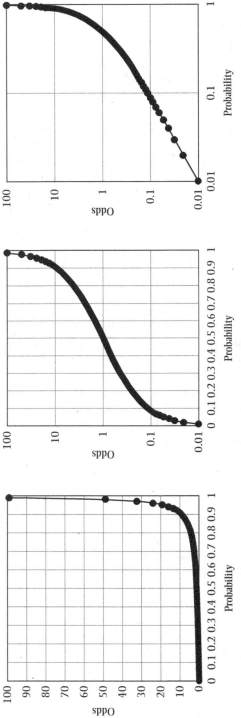

Figure 1.1 The relationship between prevalence proportion and prevalence odds, or more generally (and as it is labeled) between probability and odds. Left panel shows natural scales for both axes, middle panel shows natural scale for the probability and $\log_{10}$ scale for the odds, right panel shows $\log_{10}$ scale for the probability and $\log_{10}$ scale for the odds. Left panel shows natural scales for both.

Box 1.2

Incidence Proportion, Risks, and "Risk Factors"

Incidence proportion and "risk" are sometimes used interchangeably in epidemiology, and we use risk as a synonym for incidence proportion here (although incidence proportion is less ambiguous). It is worth, however, parsing out "risk factor" as another term that is frequently used in epidemiologic investigations but which is far less clear. Sometimes "risk factor" means "a cause of disease," and sometimes it merely means "something whose presence is associated with an increased risk (or rate, or prevalence, or odds, or hazard) of disease, but which may or may not be a cause." The difference between these two usages will become clearer in the next chapters.

Prevalence counts are sometimes useful in communicating the public health importance of a disease condition or in contexts where incidence is difficult to define and so you want to have a sense of numbers of events for surveillance purposes. Unfortunately, prevalence counts are just as often used to overhype that importance by reporting large-sounding numbers without appropriate context. Prevalence counts are therefore of most use when their context is well-understood by the audience: for example, since most residents of the United States have a general sense of the total population of that country, a report to a US audience of the prevalence count of US residents living with COPD (at this writing, about 13 million) might be adequately contextualized.

As with all counts, the prevalence count is an integer between 0 however many possible cases exist in the population being examined. For a recurrent event measured over a sufficiently long period of time (e.g., upper respiratory infections), the prevalence count might exceed the number of individuals in the population: however, in such a case, calculating an incidence might be more straightforward.

1.2 INCIDENCE

Where prevalence is a measure of how many cases of disease or condition are present at a given moment or over a period, *incidence* is a measure of how many *new cases of a disease arise over a specified period of time*. A critical difference between prevalence and incidence is that, unlike prevalence, incidence is a measure of occurrences, or events: incidence counts the number of transitions from a condition being absent in an individual to that condition being present.

We can measure the incidence of both one-time events (incidence of Parkinson's disease or incidence of first cancer diagnosis) and recurrent events (number of respiratory infections in a calendar year). Thus, to measure incidence, we must start from a population at risk of the disease outcome: for example, to measure the incidence of Parkinson's disease in our cohort, we must not include people who already have Parkinson's disease at cohort inception. It is important to note that we can turn a recurrent event into a one-time event by restricting our study to the first occurrence of that event: for example, first respiratory infection for each individual in the calendar year.

We measure incidence in many of the same ways as we measure prevalence: as incidence proportions, incidence odds, and incidence counts (i.e., counts of new cases of disease in a population). In addition, we use incidence rates and measures of elapsed time to an event. All of these measures, however, can be productively viewed as derivations, or simplifications, of a survival curve or cumulative incidence curve. Thus, we discuss the survival curve.

1.2.1 Survival and the Survival Curve

Survival, it has been argued, is the core measure of public health because health outcomes in a population typically occur over time.[2] The most unambiguous health outcome is death (the one incident outcome which—by convention—we never describe as prevalent). Here we consider timing of death for any reason, an example termed "all-cause mortality" and chosen for its simplicity. Date of death can often be measured without appreciable error (due to death records—although cause of death is a different story); death is a one-time event; death ultimately will affect everyone.

We start with 1,000 30-year-olds in the imaginary city of Calvino: at the moment they turn 30, all 1,000 are alive. By age 35, 30 of those individuals have died; by age 40, another 40 have died, leaving 930 Calvinians alive. By age 90, all 1,000 of these 30-year-olds have died.

How would we collect such data? Suppose we begin studying 1,000 individuals who are 30 years old: all these participants are living, and our study continues until they have all died. We collect numbers of those individuals who have died every 5 years, generating data as shown in Table 1.1.

How would we depict the data in Table 1.1 visually? Two methods are widely used: the *Kaplan-Meier method* and the *life table method*, both of which are described in detail in Chapter 5, when we apply these methods to analysis of randomized trial data. Here we show a modified Kaplan-Meier approach for tabled data.

We can draw a survival curve, or cumulative incidence curve, for these data by placing points for each number surviving (Figure 1.2, left) and then connecting these with a step function (Figure 1.2, right). We use a step function to indicate that we only know what happens every 5 years: for example, at age 35 there were 970 participants still alive, and the next piece of information we have is that at

---

2. Although time is irrelevant, or nearly so, in counting deaths from certain natural disasters such as earthquakes.

Table 1.1 SAMPLE DATA OF 1,000 30-
YEAR-OLDS FOLLOWED UNTIL DEATH

Age	Number surviving
30	1,000
35	970
40	930
45	880
50	820
55	750
60	670
65	560
70	460
75	350
80	230
85	100
90	0

age 40 there were only 930 participants still alive. In between those times we do not know what happened, and thus we only update our curve when we acquire new information. Note that we could also draw a cumulative incidence curve here in which a curve starts at 0 and rises toward 100% as cases accumulate (Cole & Hudgens, 2010; Pocock, Clayton, & Altman, 2002).

What we have described is a (very) special case of the Kaplan-Meier curve. The Kaplan-Meier curve is formally defined for data collected in continuous time (i.e., exactly how old was each individual when they died?) and such a curve can account for individuals who go missing during follow-up (and are "censored"). Again, we give more detail on the Kaplan-Meier curve (and the alternative life table method, which does not assume a step function) in Chapter 5.

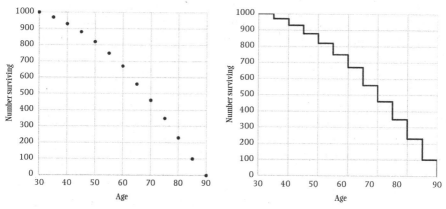

Figure 1.2 Graphical displays of data shown in Table 1.1.

1.2.2 Incidence Proportion (Risk)

Incidence proportion, a phrase we use interchangeably with "risk" in this work, is defined as the proportion of those at study inception who are capable of experiencing the outcome (sometimes called the population "at risk") and who experience an outcome in a fixed period of time. Incidence proportion is bounded between 0 (no one experiences the outcome) and 1 (all those at risk experience the outcome). Assuming outcomes are measured correctly (including accurately in time), incidence proportion can be estimated without further assumptions when all those at risk are followed for the full time period of follow-up.

Here, we indeed assume that all participants are followed for the full study period and we have outcome information on all of them (complete follow-up). In the context of the Kaplan-Meier estimator in Chapter 5, we will discuss how to calculate risks when we lose track of some study participants (e.g., they are lost to follow-up) or do not record their study outcomes for some reason (they have missing data).

Under these assumptions, however, incidence proportion can be derived directly from the survival curve—well, these assumptions and one more. The additional assumption is that all events shown happen at the last possible moment in each time interval. There are 1,000 people alive from age 30 up until the moment before age 35, and, at that last possible moment, all 30 people die at once. Similarly, until one instant before age 40, all 970 people are alive; then 40 people die, leading to 930 people alive at age 40. This is obviously not realistic![3] But it helps us illustrate our points.

In Figure 1.3, we redraw the survival curve from Figure 1.2 in terms of percentages rather than participants, and then we draw a dashed line through that curve at 40 years of age. The dotted line intersects the survival curve at 93% on the y-axis, indicating that 93% of those participants present at baseline remain alive. We can then calculate the 40-year risk of death as 1 − 93% = 7%.

In general, an incidence proportion is exactly what its name implies: the proportion of the at-risk population who experienced an outcome within a given time period. The incidence proportion can be estimated without reference to the survival curve: you could obtain the same estimate of risk as from Figure 1.2 (or the data in Table 1.1) directly, simply by observing that 930 individuals were alive at age 40, noting that this means 70 had died, and dividing 70 by the original number in the study (1,000) to get 7%.

Incidence proportions are *not* commonly thought of in terms of the underlying survival curves: in this case, as we have illustrated, no knowledge of the intervening survival curve is necessary to estimate the 40-year risk. But it is still the underlying survival curve which is the better description of the shape of survival in these participants. In Figure 1.4, for example, the new data shown are all consistent with a 20% incidence proportion (80% survival) at age 40 but all three are different. On

---

3. In reality, the 30 people who have died between ages 30 and 35 all died at some intermediate point in that interval—probably at a rate increasing with age—so more died at 34 than at 31. If this is true—but we only see the deaths at the end of the interval—we consider the deaths to be *interval censored*. That is, we know they happened between ages 30 and 35, but we don't know when.

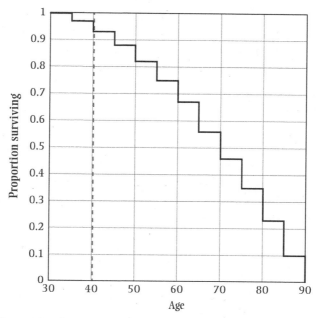

Figure 1.3 Figure 1.2 redrawn using percentages instead of counts.

the left, the deaths occur equally before and after age 35; in the center, the deaths occur mostly after age 35; and, on the right, the deaths occur mostly before age 35. If you were a 30-year-old to whom these figures applied (if, for example, these figures estimated risk of death among individuals with a deadly but treatable condition), it would likely matter a great deal to you which of these three figures represented the truth: an incidence proportion of 20% doesn't give you this information.

It is critical to reiterate that incidence proportions are only meaningful when paired with a fixed period of time. This may be illustrated most clearly with the outcome of death: the "risk of death" in humans is universally 1, in that all humans will eventually die. Thus, telling someone that, in your study, the "risk of death was 10%" is unhelpful; more helpful would be to tell them that, for example, the "1-year risk of death was 10%." It is more difficult to state such a risk clearly when length of follow-up is reasonably well-defined and yet differs by time scale: for

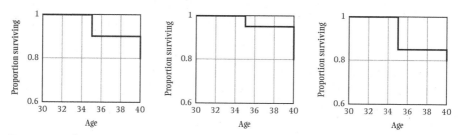

Figure 1.4 Three curves, all showing the same cumulative incidence of death by age 40.

example, people discuss the "lifetime risk" of cancer or depression, but such risks strongly depend on how long you live. Likewise, risk of infection during a hospital stay may not be well-defined when length of stay varies, but may nonetheless be a useful measure to discuss.

1.2.3 Incidence Odds

The relationship of incidence odds to incidence proportion is precisely the same mathematical relationship as that of prevalence odds to prevalence proportion (though incidence odds seem to be estimated less often in practice than prevalence odds). If the 30-day incidence proportion of hospital readmission following a first myocardial infarction was 20%, then the 30-day incidence odds would be $0.20/(1.00 - 0.20) = 0.25$. You can easily generalize further details from the preceding section on prevalence odds however like incidence proportions, incidence odds require a set period of time. But, as with prevalence odds, for example, the incidence odds ranges from 0 to infinity (and Figure 1.1 may again be useful).

The derivation of the incidence odds from the survival curve is likewise straightforward. Consider Figure 1.3 again and death at age 40 among those who started follow-up. Rather than taking $1.00 - 0.93$ to get an incidence proportion of 0.07 at age 40, we would now take the ratio of distance above the curve (0.07) to distance below the curve (0.93) and get $0.07/0.93 = 0.0753$. Note that, in line with the "10% rule of thumb" given in Box 1.1, the odds here is not too far from the risk of 0.07. See also Box 1.3.

1.2.4 Incidence Rate

As noted earlier (Figure 1.4), incidence proportions can obscure differences between two groups over time. Look at the two survival curves in Figure 1.5,

---

Box 1.3

SLIM TO NONE

"The odds are slim to none" is a phrase in occasional usage and is meant to indicate a small probability. But it is misleading if taken literally. Suppose we take a "slim" probability to be 1 in 100; then "the odds are slim to none" (slim:none) literally means that the odds is calculated by dividing the probability of slim by the probability of none, or $(1/100)/0$. We calculate, of course, an infinite odds (or perhaps one which is undefined). Thus, the cliché, taken literally, yields precisely the opposite of its intended meaning, wherein "the odds are slim to none" means in fact that the odds are extremely (infinitely!) high. "The chances are slim to none," on the other hand, conveys the intended meaning without sacrificing accuracy.

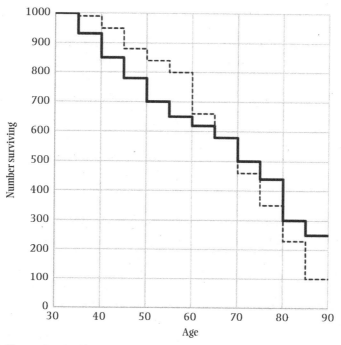

Figure 1.5 Illustrating incidence rates using two survival curves.

one solid, one dotted (note that we have shifted our y-axis back to counts of people rather than percentages). Each curve represents a group of 1,000 participants. While the two curves cross at 65 years of age, they are fairly different until that point: the dotted curve stays high until age 60 and then dips sharply, while the solid curve declines more steadily over time. The curves clearly represent different experiences of mortality, and the area under the curves might well be different—but, nonetheless, at age 65 the incidence proportions are identical.

We might wonder whether there is a way to summarize these two curves that preserves the differences between them. There are several: here, we concentrate on the *incidence rate*. The incidence rate is a measure of the average intensity at which an event occurs in the experience of people over time, and, for a population followed from baseline, it is calculated as the *number of cases* in that population divided by the *amount of person-time* at risk accumulated by that population.

Person-time is the amount of time observed for all people under study while at risk of experiencing an incident outcome: if a woman is followed for 1 month, then she experiences (and contributes to analysis) 1 person-month of time. If 10 women are followed for 1 year, they contribute 10 × 1 = 10 person-years; if 1 woman is followed for 10 years, she also contributes 1 × 10 = 10 person-years. This

Table 1.2 CALCULATION OF RISKS AND RATES FOR DATA SHOWN IN FIGURE 1.5

	Total at age 30	Events by age 65	Person-time by age 65	Incidence rate[a] from ages 30 to 65	Risk at age 65
Solid line	1,000	420	30,550	1.37	42%
Dotted line	1,000	420	33,500	1.25	42%

[a]Incidence rate given in deaths per 100 person-years.

calls attention to a basic assumption of person-time: that any unit of person-time is exchangeable with any other unit of person-time under study.[4]

How do we calculate the incidence rate from the curves shown in Figure 1.5? In both curves the numerator is the number of cases; in both situations the denominator is the amount of person-time accumulated to that point—in this case, we'll consider the incidence rates until age 65. Conceptually, that person-time can be calculated: because the y-axis is measured by a count of people, person-time for each incidence rate is simply the area under each survival curve. In this case, the dotted line has accumulated person-time of 33,500 person-years, the solid line has accumulated person-time of 30,550 person-years. The incidence rates are calculated in Table 1.2. We see that the incidence rate for the outcome is higher for the solid line. Thus, while being in the solid versus dotted group seems to give you an equal chance of surviving until age 65, you may nonetheless live longer (e.g., die later in that interval) if you are in the dotted group.

Unlike the incidence proportion, the incidence rate does not need to be reported with a specific time period attached[5]; for example, the incidence rate in the dotted cohort could be reported with or without the bracketed statement: "the incidence rate of death in the dotted line group (over a period of 35 years) was 1.25 per 100 person-years." On a related topic, because person-time is flexible, incidence rates can be reported on a variety of scales. For example, note that 100 events per person-year is equivalent to 100 events per 12 person-months is equivalent to 8.33 events per person-month is equivalent to 10,000 events per 100 person-years. Because we can scale up or down the actual numbers of an incidence rate as we need to, the range of the incidence rate is 0 to infinity; in general, incidence rates should be reported on a scale appropriate or standard to the substantive context.

Two key differences between the incidence proportion and incidence rate are worth highlighting. First, consider a situation in which we have data on 10 people, each followed-up for a different length of time. In this case a straightforward risk calculation would likely be invalid: the proportion of those 10 people who

4. This is not always true, of course, and can be relaxed in practice under certain assumptions or by examining the rate as it changes over time. But it is nonetheless important.

5. Although it can and perhaps should be! You might interpret a rate differently knowing it had been measured over 1 year, 5 years, or 10 years.

experienced an outcome would not be in a fixed period of time and thus would not typically or simply be interpretable as an incidence proportion. On the other hand, we could calculate the total person-time accumulated by those individuals and use that as the denominator for an incidence rate without concern that each individual contributed a different amount of time over follow-up. However, it is important to note that this difference only applies to the risk calculation from a straightforward proportion: we could use a Kaplan-Meier estimator or other method to estimate the risk at a given point during follow-up (see Chapter 5).

Second, the incidence rates can account for *recurrent events*, whereas incidence proportions cannot. Recall that the incidence proportion is constrained to be between 0 and 1: thus, with N people, the incidence proportion may falter at fully describing the occurrence of $2N$ events (as might happen if we were studying the number of upper respiratory infections experienced by individuals over a period of 6 months). Where an incidence rate can accumulate both a count of events and an experience of cumulative person-time among study participants *and* calculate an incidence rate, the incidence proportion might be forced to study the risk of first upper respiratory infection (and then, among those who had a first upper respiratory infection, the risk of a second and then third). These are different scientific questions and might both be of interest to public health.

1.2.5 Times to Event

So far, all the summary measures of incidence (incidence proportion, odds, rate) have simplified the survival curve by putting a vertical line through the curve at a given time. Consider instead putting a *horizontal* line through the survival curve at a given percentage incidence. See in Figure 1.6, where the y-axis remains as a percentage survival, we have placed a dotted line starting at the 50th percent mark: when we extend this line to the right, we find that it intersects with the survival curve at an x-value of 70 years. This may be interpreted as follows: in this population, median time to death is 70 years. The interpretation would be complicated if the event under study was not inevitable—see competing risks, discussed later—or if the entire cohort hadn't been followed until everyone in it had experienced it (it is very rare to follow a cohort until everyone in it has had the outcome!).

Median time to event (or other percentiles in addition to the median) is an extremely useful way to describe events in time but is not widely used in the epidemiologic and biomedical literature. We will expand on this point in the next chapter, when we discuss contrasts between times to event.

1.2.6 Confusions Between Prevalence and Incidence

As noted in Box 1.4, there is substantial confusion about naming conventions of prevalence and incidence measures, and of rates, risks, and odds. We wish to point out one additional trap into which epidemiologists, and the published literature, sometimes fall. It is almost always a serious mistake to interpret a point

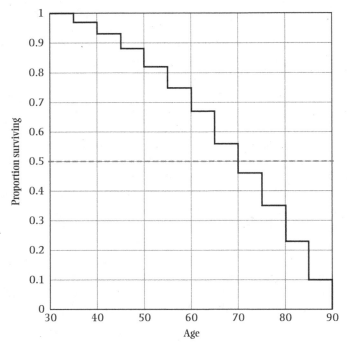

Figure 1.6 Using a survival curve to illustrate time to event.

prevalence measured after the baseline of a study (e.g., the prevalence of cancer 5 years after the start of a cohort study) as an incidence proportion. To see why this is so, consider a study in which everyone is free of depression at baseline, and the prevalence of depression (assessed in a survey of all participants) at 2 years is 20%: it is tempting (is it not?) to interpret this as the incidence of depression at 2 years. But that 20% does not consider at least two groups of people who are critical in assessing incidence: those who developed depression and then died before 2 years had elapsed and those who developed depression and then successfully treated that depression all before 2 years had elapsed.

1.2.7 Challenges in Calculating Incidence Measures

There are several key challenges in estimating the measures of incidence noted previously; we list some key challenges here, focusing on risks (incidence proportions) but also noting that some of these challenges do not apply equally to other measures of incidence. Related points are explored in greater detail in subsequent chapters.

1.2.7.1 LOSS OF PARTICIPANTS

As noted earlier, if you lose track of participants over time, you cannot know what happened to those participants in terms of the outcome under study—without

Box 1.4

Proportions, Rates, and Units

Incidence proportions are a proportion in which the numerator has the implicit unit of "cases" or "events," which can also be thought of as "people (who experienced new onset of the outcome)" and the denominator also has the unit of "people (who were at risk of the outcome)." Because people are in both the numerator and denominator, they cancel, and therefore the incidence proportion is *unitless*.

The incidence rate has a similar numerator and a denominator of *people × time*; as such, when the "people" units cancel, the incidence rate is left with units of 1 / *time*. This is why the reciprocal of the incidence rate has the unit simply "time." Relatedly, when certain conditions are met, this inverse of the incidence rate can be interpreted as the average waiting time to the event. However, it is clearer for most audiences to express incidence rates as "events per units of person-time."

Not all rates (or things which look and behave like rates) have this unit, however! For example, one can calculate a rate of traffic fatalities per 1,000 miles driven; this has the units "1/miles" rather than "1/time" but is otherwise highly analogous to incidence rates as we have described them.

Finally, numerous things are referred to as "rates" which are not in fact, rates. For example, the "unemployment rate" as it is usually described is a unitless measure of the proportion of those unemployed at a particular moment in time: a prevalence proportion, rather than a rate. The infant mortality "rate" is really a risk over the first year of life; birth defect "rates" are almost always a prevalence at live birth. The "attack rate" is generally held to mean "incidence proportion" or something similar (Porta, 2014). And, as earlier, "prevalence rate" often means "prevalence proportion" as well. Similarly, "risk" is likewise used to mean a great many things, including incidence proportion—our sole usage of "risk" in this work—but sometimes is used to mean incidence rate, hazard rate, and even prevalence.

So when you read "rate" or "risk" in popular press contexts—and even in scientific reports—take a moment to make sure you understand what measure is being discussed.

---

assumptions, then, you can't calculate risk. For example, you are studying heart attack in 100 people, and 20 people drop out of your study: of the remaining 80, 16 had heart attacks. If the study ends before all individuals have had events, resultant "administrative censoring" may present similar issues. In either case, it is tempting to calculate the risk only in those you observe, as 16/80 = 20%, and use that as your estimate of the risk of the outcome among all 100 people who started the study.

But to do so would be reasonable only if the 20 missing people looked just like the 80 non-missing people: specifically, if missingness were completely unrelated to the risk of heart attack, and therefore 4 of the missing 20 people had a heart attack. This might be true! But what if, instead, individuals who drop out are at higher than average risk of heart attack so that, in fact, 10 of the 20 missing people had a heart attack? Then the true risk would be (16 + 10)/100 or 26%. The key issue is that since these individuals are missing, you don't know whether 4, or 10, or 18, or indeed 0 of them had heart attacks, and thus taking the 16/80 as your estimate of risk among all 100 of the participants relies on possibly quite strong assumptions. Although incidence rates do not require that everyone under study is followed for the same length of time, we would likewise expect incidence rates to be biased if individuals who exit the study (and on whom we therefore lack outcome data) are systematically different from those who remain in the study.

1.2.7.2 COMPETING RISKS

Competing risks are outcomes that prevent the occurrence of the outcome under study. For example, in a study of the occurrence of cancer, death from stroke (for example) is a competing risk for the outcome in that, once a participant has died from stroke, they cannot develop cancer.

Estimating incidence proportions or other measures of incidence with survival curves and time-to-event methods under competing risks is complex and largely beyond the scope of this book. It is worth clarifying, however, that the risks estimated by the simple survival curve methods shown earlier (and throughout the remainder of this book) are all risks under the hypothetical absence of any competing risks. This is easy when the outcome is death from any cause because there are no competing risks for this outcome. In other cases, the assumption is often far less reasonable, but we may be comfortable making it if competing risks are quite rare (Cole & Hudgens, 2010).

1.2.8 Relation Between Prevalence and Incidence

Briefly, it is worth explaining how prevalence and incidence relate to each other, conceptually and mathematically. Conceptually, prevalence over a time period is a function of both incidence (how many new cases are showing up?) and duration of disease (how long does each case last?). This is because the longer the duration of disease, the more incident cases accumulate during a time period. Consider a population of 100 people, 10 of whom get an upper respiratory infection on the first day of each month. If the infection lasts a full month, then, on average, the prevalence of such infections over time will be 10%: 10/100 for the first month, then a new 10/100 for the second month. But if the infection lasts 2 months, then, after the first month, the prevalence of infection will be about 20%: 10 cases from the first month and 10 more from the second month.[6]

---

6. Or perhaps only 9 out of the remaining 90 for the second month, for a prevalence of 19%. This points toward the need to calculate cumulative incidence using more complicated methods.

This suggests a rough equivalency between prevalence, incidence, and duration, of the form

$$Prevalence \approx Incidence \times Duration$$

where the squiggly equals sign ($\approx$) means "approximately equal to." More precisely, the relationship is

$$\frac{Prevalence\ proportion}{1 - Prevalence\ proportion} = Incidence\ rate \times Average\ duration\ of\ disease$$

where the left side of the equation is exactly prevalence odds. This relationship will hold when the population is in "steady-state"; that is, constant (or nearly so) in composition and size and with constant (or nearly so) incidence rate and disease duration (Rothman, 2012; Rothman, Greenland, & Lash, 2008). If prevalence of the disease is low (typically, <10%), then this calculated prevalence odds will approximately equal to the prevalence proportion.

1.2.9 Relation Between Risk (Incidence Proportion) and Incidence Rate

In our preceding example, we might not get 10 cases in the second month: after the first month, there are only 90 people left who are not infected. If the incidence were 10% per month, we would expect 9 new cases, rather than 10, because the population at risk of infection declines over time. This points to the relationship between the incidence rate and the incidence proportion (sometimes in this context called the *cumulative incidence*). In a closed cohort with a constant incidence rate, these two measures are related by the exponential formula as follows:

$$Risk = 1 - e^{-Incidence\ rate \times Time}$$

where $e = 2.71828...$ and time is the amount of time over which we wish to estimate risk (Rothman et al., 2008). Note again that here we are assuming a closed cohort (such that the number of individuals is diminishing over time), whereas in the relationship between prevalence and incidence, we assumed a steady-state population (people who leave the cohort are replaced by people entering the cohort). However, in parallel to the preceding relationship between prevalence and incidence, when risk is <10%, this relationship can be estimated as

$$Risk \approx Incidence\ rate \times Time.$$

1.3 SYSTEMATIC AND RANDOM ERROR

Now, having discussed some preliminary measures but before making our way to contrasts (Chapter 2), a brief word on *systematic error* and *random error*. The simplest way to explain the difference between random error and systematic error is that random error gets smaller as your sample size increases; systematic error does not.

Suppose you are tossing a coin and you want to know whether it is "fair" or not: you want to know whether the probability of the coin coming up heads is 50% (which we'll call "unbiased"). If you flip a fair coin (fairly!) 10 times, there's a pretty good chance that you will get 3 or fewer heads, even though the coin is indeed fair: specifically, the probability is about 17% that you'll get 3, 2, 1, or 0 heads. But after 1,000 flips with a truly fair coin, it is quite unlikely that you'll wind up with 300 or fewer heads (specifically, the probability is <0.00001). With a truly fair coin (flipped fairly!), the reason you do not always get exactly 5 heads out of 10 flips is random error—in general, the more times you flip the coin the closer your number of heads will probably be to half the number of times you flipped the coin: after 1,000 flips of a fair coin, the probability is 89% that you wind up with between 475 and 525 heads. (Although it is important to note that the chances you'll get exactly 500 heads is extremely small.)

Systematic error, in this example, might be seen as the case in which the coin is, in fact, not fair. Suppose that the probability of the coin coming up heads is 70%: in 1,000 coin flips, the chances you get a value between 475 and 525 is now likewise <0.00001—but there's a >90% probability that you'll have between 675 and 725 heads.

Frequently, we call random error "variance" (and we often call the *lack* of random error "precision"); we call systematic error "bias" (and *lack* of such bias "validity"). Numbers we care about in epidemiology (e.g., the risk of some disease) can be estimated with high precision and high validity, low precision and low validity, or some combination of those factors. The bulls-eye representations in Figure 1.7 are often used to introduce topics of precision and validity in epidemiology textbooks. Figure 1.7 shows all four combinations of low/high precision and validity in attempting to pinpoint ("estimate") the center of the figure. In the lower right box, we show an estimation approach with high precision (tight clustering of points) and high validity (they cluster around the true center). In the upper right box, we still have high precision/low validity (tight clustering, but points are not near the true center). In the lower left box, we have low precision/high validity (loose clustering, and, while it is hard to see, the points are on average around the true center). And in the upper left box, we have low precision/low validity (loose clustering, not around the true center).

The difference between random error and systematic error is in some sense the difference between a first course in biostatistics and a first course in epidemiology: while of course epidemiologists are concerned with random error as well as systematic error, and biostatisticians vice versa, the broad domains of the disciplines at their introductory levels are somewhat captured in this distinction.

Low precision   High precision

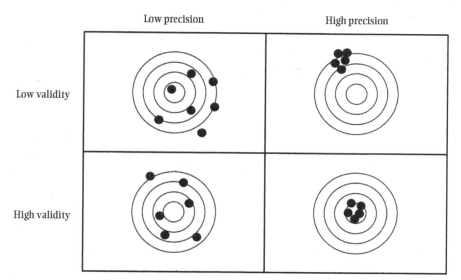

Low validity

High validity

Figure 1.7 Precision and validity.

As such, this book—a first text in epidemiology—is concerned near exclusively with systematic error. In this work, we will primarily concentrate on systematic error and in trying to estimate quantities (risk differences, risk ratios, and so on) with minimal bias (systematic error). Perhaps, as one reviewer of this text suggested, it is more accurate but less efficient to say that, in this work, we will (1) try to understand how to estimate quantities while reducing bias as much as possible, (2) while paying attention to both direction and magnitude of the bias that will likely if not inevitably remain, (3) while bearing in mind the complex relationship between validity and precision in that we can sometimes increase one while reducing the other. We will not, in this work, overly focus on the precision (random error, variance) of those estimates, though we will not ignore issues of random error either. We address related topics of p-values and 95% confidence limits in Chapter 5 when discussing randomized trials.

REFERENCES

Bland, J. M., & Altman, D. G. (2000). Statistics notes. The odds ratio. *British Medical Journal, 320*(7247), 1468.

Cole, S. R., & Hudgens, M. G. (2010). Survival analysis in infectious disease research: Describing events in time. *AIDS, 24*(16), 2423–2431. doi:10.1097/QAD.0b013e32833dd0ec

Greenland, S. (1987). Interpretation and choice of effect measures in epidemiologic analyses. *American Journal of Epidemiology, 125*(5), 761–768.

Pocock, S. J., Clayton, T. C., & Altman, D. G. (2002). Survival plots of time-to-event outcomes in clinical trials: Good practice and pitfalls. *Lancet, 359*(9318), 1686–1689. doi:10.1016/S0140-6736(02)08594-X

Porta, M. (Ed.). (2014). *A dictionary of epidemiology* (6th ed.). New York: Oxford University Press.

Rothman, K. J. (2012). *Epidemiology: An introduction.* New York: Oxford University Press.

Rothman, K. J., Greenland, S., & Lash, T. L. (2008). *Modern epidemiology* (3rd ed.). Philadelphia: Lippincott Williams & Wilkins.

2

Measures of Association

In the previous chapter, we discussed how to describe a single cohort, alluding to differences between groups within that cohort only to illustrate the need for additional measures of description. Here, we discuss several ways that one can compare the risks of an outcome in two distinct groups, perhaps groups defined by exposures or treatments. We will also discuss how to communicate these findings for researchers, policy makers, clinicians, and patients, all of whom may need to make decisions based on such comparisons.

2.1 OVERVIEW

In this chapter, we describe summary measures of association, among them risk differences and ratios, odds ratios, incidence rate ratios, and time differences and ratios. After describing these measures and how to calculate them, we discuss how to choose among these measures: the advantages and disadvantages of each measure compared to the others. While our focus here is on associations between measures of incidence (e.g., risks/incidence proportions), many of the points in this chapter may also be applied to measures of prevalence (e.g., prevalence proportions). In addition, associations may be interpretable as causal effects under certain conditions (see Chapter 3).

As we showed in Chapter 1, the components of these measures of association and impact—the risks (incidence proportions) and incidence rates and times to event—can be derived from the survival curve. As such, comparisons of two risks can likewise be derived from two survival curves. Comparison of two survival curves as a whole—that is, without summarizing them into incidence proportions or incidence rates or median times to event—is also possible, though we defer discussion to Chapter 5.

Outcomes in this chapter will typically be dichotomous (having two categories), such as "alive or dead," or "diseased or not-diseased," or "outcome or no outcome." We do not address continuous outcomes much in this chapter, such as "weight lost or gained" or "inches of height grown" in a set period of time. The one place where we do address a continuous outcome is when discussing time differences and time ratios: survival time (or time until some event occurs) is a continuous

Epidemiology by Design: A Causal Approach to the Health Sciences. Daniel Westreich, Oxford University Press (2020). © Oxford University Press.
DOI: 10.1093/oso/9780190665760.001.0001

outcome. Many concepts presented in this chapter can be generalized to other continuous outcomes such as weight.

2.2 SUMMARY MEASURES OF ASSOCIATION

2.2.1 Null Values

Before we describe any measures of association or how to calculate them, we need to first define the idea of a *null value* in a measure of association (or causal effect, see Chapter 3). The null value of a measure of association is *the value that measure takes when there is no difference between the two groups being compared*. When the risk of the outcome is the same in exposed and unexposed groups, we should expect contrasts of those risks to have the null value. We define null values for each major measure of association described here.

2.2.2 The 2 × 2 Table

While comparing two survival curves as a whole can be extremely useful, it is also often desirable to summarize the survival curves such that a more compact comparison can be made. Accordingly, many of the contrast measures in this chapter (risk differences, risk ratios, odds ratios, and others) will rely on explanations and illustrations from 2 × 2 tables—a central tool in the teaching of epidemiologic methods.

Consider a hypothetical study in which a cohort of disease-free individuals was followed for 5 years, with no loss of participants and no competing risks (see Chapter 1, "Challenges in Calculating Incidence Measures"). We are studying some health outcome of interest, for example, occurrence of first heart attack. In Table 2.1, we show a table describing such a study for two exposure categories, exposed ($X = 1$) and unexposed ($X = 0$). The table also shows two outcome categories—those who experienced a heart attack by the end of follow-up ($Y = 1$) and those who did not experience it ($Y = 0$). For the moment, we notate the combinations of X and Y as A, B, C, D, each of which is a count of people. We read from this as follows: of the $A + B$ people who were exposed ($X = 1$), A experienced

Table 2.1 A GENERIC 2 × 2 TABLE

	$Y = 1$ (Experienced outcome)	$Y = 0$ (No outcome)	Total
$X = 1$ (Exposed)	A	B	$A + B$
$X = 0$ (Not exposed)	C	D	$C + D$
Total	$A + C$	$B + D$	$A + B + C + D$

Note: if the axes are reversed (with Outcomes on the rows, and Exposure on the columns) that the calculations below will not work as intended.

the outcome ($Y = 1$) and B did not ($Y = 0$). Of the $C + D$ people who were unexposed ($X = 0$), C experienced the outcome ($Y = 1$) and D did not ($Y = 0$).

If all the subjects have their exposure and outcome measured at the same moment in time, we could use this table to calculate the proportions of those exposed and unexposed who have the outcome and thus perhaps understand issues related to cross-sectional disease prevalence. On the other hand, if we know (or assume) that exposure was measured at the beginning of some follow-up period and that all $A + B + C + D$ subjects were followed-up for the same length of time and then had their outcome assessed, then we could use these data to calculate incidence proportions or an incidence odds in the exposed and separately unexposed individuals.

As we discussed in Chapter 1, the incidence proportion may be frequently preferable to the incidence odds because the incidence odds will tend to overstate the incidence proportion when outcomes are common; nonetheless calculating the incidence odds ratio is sometimes desirable (see the discussion of logistic regression in Chapter 6). In Table 2.1, we can calculate the incidence proportion among the exposed participants as simply

$$A / (A + B)$$

representing the statement that, of $A + B$ total exposed people, A experienced the outcome. Among the unexposed participants, the incidence proportion is simply $C/(C + D)$. The incidence odds among the exposed is calculated as

$$(A / (A + B)) / (1 - (A / (A + B)))$$

which simplifies to A/B; among the unexposed, the incidence odds are likewise C/D. Later, we provide examples in discussing measures of association. It is critical to note that if the axes of Table 2.1 were reversed—such that Outcomes were read across rows, and Exposures were read down columns—these calculations would not give the correct answers.

In general, all the measures that will be described in the remainder of the chapter can be safely interpreted as measures of association (or *contrast*). To interpret them as measures of *causal effect* (or, sometimes, *effect* or *impact*) requires additional assumptions (to be discussed in Chapter 3).

2.2.3 The Risk Difference

The risk difference, which is occasionally called the *incidence proportion difference*, is calculated directly from the data presented in a 2 × 2 table. Consider an example, Table 2.2, in which we follow people who are free of cancer at the beginning of follow-up, after an environmental disaster which exposed some of them to a particular environmental contaminant. We enroll 2,000 individuals

Table 2.2 A 2 × 2 TABLE FOR THE ASSOCIATION OF
EXPOSURE TO AN ENVIRONMENTAL CONTAMINANT
AND 5-YEAR CANCER RISK

	Cancer	No cancer	Total	Risk
Exposed	70	930	1,000	0.070
Unexposed	30	970	1,000	0.030
Total	100	1,900	2,000	

from the affected area and take measurements of exposure in these individuals. We find that 1,000 are exposed, and 1,000 are unexposed. We follow these 2,000 participants for 5 years to determine who in each group develops a new cancer in that period. Suppose that 70 of the exposed participants developed cancer, and 30 of those who were not exposed also developed cancer.

Using this information, we can complete the 2 × 2 table as follows, recalling that this 2 × 2 is a *summary* of two curves of cancer-free survival over time. Here, it is straightforward to calculate the 5-year risk of cancer in exposed and (separately) unexposed study participants. In exposed participants, 5-year risk is 70/1000, or 7%; in the unexposed, 5-year risk is 30/1000, or 3%. The *risk difference* is simply the difference between those two risks: 7% − 3%, or 4%. We can express this risk difference in words as follows: "The 5-year risk difference comparing study participants exposed to the contaminant to those who were unexposed was 4%."

What does this mean in reality? One further interpretation is: for every 1,000 persons who are observed to be exposed to the contaminant (and if those people resemble those we studied), we would expect to likewise observe an additional 40 new cancer cases above the background cancer rate over 5 years.[1]

A critical point: the risk difference calculated from a 2 × 2 table is interpretable only if all participants under study are followed for the same length of time. For example, it might well be misleading to compare risk of cancer evaluated at 3 years in some exposed participants with risk at 5 years in some unexposed participants. That said, in practice, we often let small differences in follow-up time slide; alternatively, we could calculate a difference in incidence rates, which naturally accounts for different amounts of person-time (see later discussion). Furthermore, it is possible to calculate a risk difference in a population with heterogeneous follow-up times; see, for example, the Kaplan-Meier approach described in Chapter 5. However, even using such an approach, it is critical to specify the period of time in which the risk difference applies when stating or interpreting a risk difference. We talk further about how to discuss risk differences and risk ratios in Box 2.1.

Several somewhat technical points about the risk difference measure should be called out here. First, the range of the risk difference is from −1 to +1, inclusive (which we express as [−1, 1]). This is because the highest possible risk is 1, while the

---

1. Note, again, that this interpretation does not specifically claim that the additional cancer cases were *caused* by exposure to the contaminant: such a claim would require substantial additional assumptions to be made (see Chapter 3).

Box 2.1

AMBIGUITIES IN STATING THE RISK DIFFERENCE AND RISK RATIO

Clear communication about risk difference and risk ratios can be more difficult than is sometimes thought.

A common way of expressing an association is "The 5-year risk in the exposed was 10% higher than the 5-year risk in the unexposed." The problem with this statement is that "10% higher" can be reasonably interpreted to mean either "a risk difference of 10%," as in risk in the unexposed is 20% and in the exposed is 30%. But the same phrase can be reasonably interpreted to mean "a risk ratio of 1.1," as in risk in the unexposed is 20% and in the exposed is 22% (22 is 10% higher than 20). Obviously, in this case, the two interpretations imply qualitatively different things about the risk in the exposed; thus, clarity is extremely important. There are several clearer ways to express these thoughts. To express the risk difference, the easiest thing to do is to include words like "difference" or "absolute scale" in your statements; for example, "the 5-year risk difference was 10% higher on the absolute scale" or "the 5-year absolute difference in risk was 10%" or "we would expect to observe 10 more cases per 100 people over 5 years" or "the 5-year risk in the exposed was 10 percentage points higher than the unexposed." Some of these phrases are clunky, but they are all less ambiguous than "10% higher."

Risk ratios can be expressed similarly, as in "the 5-year risk ratio comparing the exposed to the unexposed was 1.1" or "the 5-year risk in the exposed was 1.1 times that in the unexposed." In the latter example, note that "1.1 times the risk" is unambiguous, while the phrasing "1.1 times higher than" has problems similar to a statement like "the risk increased 100%," and so can leave readers confused as to whether the risk ratio being described is 1.1 or 2.1.

lowest is 0; if, as in Table 2.2, the risk in the exposed is higher than in the unexposed, then the risk cannot be higher than $1 - 0 = 1$. Similarly, when the risk in the exposed is lower than in the unexposed, then the risk cannot be lower than $0 - 1 = -1$. A negative risk difference would occur if the exposure was protective; for instance, if we were considering the association of daily aspirin use with risk of heart attack. Whether the exposure is associated with increased or decreased risk, the risk difference is considered relative to the *null value*. Again, this is the value which reflects *no differences between the two groups being compared*. No differences here would mean that the risk in exposed participants and the risk in unexposed participants are the same value P. Therefore, the null for the risk difference is $P - P = 0$.

2.2.4 The Risk Ratio

The risk (incidence proportion) ratio can be calculated straightforwardly from the information in Table 2.2: the ratio between the two risks is $0.07/0.03 = 7\%/3\% = 2.33$. One way to express this risk ratio in words is as follows: "The 5-year risk ratio comparing exposed to unexposed study participants is 2.33." Alternatively, we could say that "Over 5 years, we would expect to see 2.33 times the incidence of cancer among exposed study participants compared to unexposed study participants." More discussion can be found in Box 2.1.

In general when the risk in the exposed and unexposed is the same, the risk ratio is $P/P = 1$, which is its null value. One exception occurs when the risk is zero in both groups, in which case the risk ratio is undefined. As with the risk difference, we define the range of the risk ratio by considering the extreme cases of the risks: when the risk in the exposed is 0 and in the unexposed is any value greater than 0, the risk ratio is 0. When the risk in the exposed is any value greater than 0, then, as the risk in the unexposed approaches zero, the risk ratio approaches infinity. Thus, the range of the risk ratio is from 0 to infinity. When the risk among the exposed is lower than among the unexposed, the risk ratio will sit between 0 and 1; for example, if the risk among the exposed were half that among the unexposed, the risk ratio would be 0.5.

Unlike the risk difference, which has a symmetric range from -1 to 1, the risk ratio has an *asymmetric* range around its null value: from 0 to 1 below the null, but 1 to infinity above the null. This can sometimes present a challenge: a risk ratio of 3 may look more impressive than a risk ratio of 0.25, but a risk ratio of 0.25 is a larger magnitude of association than 3. There are two easy ways to compare the magnitude of an association above the null and below the null. The first, and simpler, is to take the reciprocal of the value below the null: in this case, the reciprocal of 0.25 is $1/0.25 = 4$. Since 4 is greater in magnitude than 3, we conclude that 0.25 is of a larger magnitude (further away from the null) than 3.

An alternative approach is to compare the absolute values of the natural log of each risk ratio: if we take $\ln(3) \sim = 1.10$ and the $\ln(0.25) \sim = -1.39$, we see that $|-1.39| > |1.10|$ and come to the same conclusion as the preceding. On the natural log-scale, the null value of the risk ratio is $\ln(1) = 0$ and the values of the log-risk ratio are symmetric around that null value of 0. For this reason, the risk ratio is sometimes graphed or shown on the log-scale.

2.2.5 The Incidence Odds Ratio

Working off the same 2×2 table, we could calculate the incidence odds ratio (often just "the odds ratio") as the ratio of the odds of cancer given exposure and the odds of cancer given nonexposure.

The odds of cancer given exposure can be calculated from Table 2.3 in several ways, including

$0.07/(1-0.07) = 0.07/0.93 = 0.075$, or $70/1000 / (1 - 70/1000) = 70/930 = 0.075$; odds of cancer among unexposed participants can be calculated in a comparable manner (and are 0.031). The odds ratio of the exposed to the unexposed $0.075/0.031$ is 2.43. The odds ratio can be reported similarly to the risk ratio, for example "The 5-year odds of cancer in exposed participants was 2.43 times the 5-year odds in unexposed participants."

Table 2.3 A 2 × 2 TABLE FOR THE ASSOCIATION OF EXPOSURE
VERSUS NONEXPOSURE ON 5-YEAR CANCER RISK,
WITH CALCULATED RISKS AND ODDS

	Cancer	No cancer	Total	Risk	Odds
Exposed	70	930	1,000	0.070	0.075
Unexposed	30	970	1,000	0.030	0.031
Total	100	1,900	2,000		

Unless you are a serious sports gambler, the odds are that you do not have a good sense of what "odds" really means—except for a general sense that it means something like "chance" or "likelihood" or "probability." And this is the key drawback of the odds ratio in its most common usage: it is very hard to intuitively interpret the odds ratio except as an approximation of the risk ratio, in much the same way that it is hard to interpret the odds except as an approximation of the risk (Chapter 1). Compounding this interpretive difficulty is that whenever the risk ratio is above the null (higher than 1), the odds ratio will be further from the null than the risk ratio. Likewise, if the risk ratio is below the null, the odds ratio will likewise be further from the null. When the absolute risks in each exposure group are high (whether or not the risk ratio itself is high), the odds ratio may substantially overstate the risk ratio. For example, when the risk in the unexposed is 30% and the risk in the exposed is 60%, the risk ratio is 0.60/0.30 = 2, and the odds ratio is $(0.60/(1 - 0.60)) / (0.30/(1 - 0.30)) = 3.5$—a substantial overstatement of the risk ratio of 2. For additional examples, see Table 2.4, comparing the risk ratio and odds ratio in the two rightmost columns over a range of risks in the unexposed and risk ratios. However, when the risks in the two exposure groups are the same, then the odds must also be the same in the two groups. Thus, the odds ratio, like the risk ratio, has a null value of 1.

Table 2.4 RELATIONSHIP BETWEEN RISK IN THE UNEXPOSED
AND RISK DIFFERENCE, RISK RATIO, AND ODDS RATIO WITH A VERY
HIGH RISK IN THE EXPOSED

Risk in unexposed	Risk in exposed	Risk difference	Risk ratio	Odds ratio
0.00	0.99	0.99	Undefined or ∞	Undefined or ∞
0.01	0.99	0.98	99	9,801
0.05	0.99	0.94	19.8	1,881
0.10	0.99	0.89	9.9	891
0.20	0.99	0.79	4.95	396
0.40	0.99	0.59	2.475	148.5
0.75	0.99	0.24	1.32	33
0.90	0.99	0.09	1.1	11
0.98	0.99	0.01	1.01	2.02

Given these drawbacks, why would we estimate an odds ratio instead of a risk ratio? We might estimate an odds ratio if we only have the appropriate data to estimate an odds ratio (as in certain types of case-control study designs; see Chapter 7). Or, we might estimate an odds ratio because that measure is easier to estimate for statistical reasons. For example, logistic regression is a reliable and well-understood statistical approach which estimates odds ratio directly. An alternative approach, estimating the risk ratio directly, typically relies on log-binomial regression: this method is often considered less reliable, and is less widely known and taught, than logistic regression.

Like the risk ratio, the odds ratio has a range of 0 to infinity. However, the range of the odds ratio is less constrained than the risk ratio. In particular, regardless of risk in the unexposed, the odds ratio always has an upper range of infinity. Because R_E is bounded at 1, the risk difference and the risk ratio are bounded for any given R_U. For example, when R_U is 20%, then the largest possible risk ratio is $1.0/0.2 = 5$, and the largest possible risk difference is $1.0 - 0.20 = 0.80$. However, as the exposed risk R_E approaches 1, the exposed odds O_E approach infinity. As a result, for any noninfinite risk in the unexposed, R_U, $\lim_{R_E \to 1} \frac{O_E}{O_U} = \infty$. In Table 2.4, we show how the risk difference, risk ratio, and odds ratio change with a very high risk in the exposed (0.99) and an increasing risk in the unexposed (from 0.00 to 0.98).

Despite the difficulty in interpretation and the fact that (when not equal to the null) odds ratios will always be further away from the null than risk ratios, nonetheless odds ratio can be useful at times. The odds ratio will return in our discussion of the case-control study (Chapter 7): though we note here (and not for the last time!) that the odds ratio that we calculate from a case-control study is only sometimes, and not always, a direct estimate of the incidence odds ratio.

2.2.6 Incidence Rate Differences and Ratios

Just as the risk difference is the difference of two risks and the risk ratio is a ratio of two risks, so, too, the incidence rate difference is the difference of two incidence rates and the incidence rate ratio the ratio of two incidence rates. Like the risk ratio, the incidence rate ratio ranges from 0 to infinity. The incidence rate difference maintains the same "per unit of person-time" units as individual incidence rates, while the incidence rate ratio is unitless: G cases/person-time-unit divided by H cases/person-time-unit simply equals G/H, with no units attached.

As an example, we have taken the data from Table 2.3 and created likely person-time data corresponding with the exposed and unexposed groups from Table 2.3. Specifically, we assumed that those who did not get cancer experienced the full 5 years of follow-up time, while we assumed that those who developed cancer did so around year 2.5,[2] after which they stopped contributing exposed person-time. Thus, we supposed that the number of person-years experienced in the exposed

---

2. In reality, of course, it is not always true that those who get the outcome do so at the halfway point of follow-up, but it is a convenient fiction for our purposes.

Table 2.5 A 2 × 2 TABLE FOR THE ASSOCIATION OF EXPOSURE VERSUS
NONEXPOSURE ON 5-YEAR CANCER RISK, WITH PERSON-YEARS AND
CALCULATED INCIDENCE RATES

	Cancer	No cancer	Person-years	Incidence rate *per 5 person-years*
Exposed	70	930	4,825	0.0725
Unexposed	30	970	4,925	0.0305
Total	100	1,900	2,000	

group was 930 * 5 + 70 * 2.5 = 4,825 and in the unexposed group was 970 * 5 +
30 * 2.5 = 4,925. We then calculated the incidence rates per person-year as 70/
4825 in the exposed and 30/4925 in the unexposed, yielding rates of 0.0145 per
person-year and 0.0061 per person-year, respectively. We then multiplied each incidence rate by 5 to obtain the incidence rates for 5 person-years; these are shown
in Table 2.5.

Box 2.2

RELATIONS AMONG RISK, ODDS, AND INCIDENCE RATES

Comparing Table 2.3 and Table 2.5, note that, among the exposed, the numerical
value of the 5-year incidence rate (0.0725) is larger than the risk (0.070) but smaller
than the odds (0.075). The same is true for the unexposed. The reasons for this are
worth exploring, to build intuition about the risk, incidence rate, and odds.

Recall that the risk includes all subjects present at the start of follow-up in
the denominator of the risk. As such, we can think of the risk as a kind of incidence rate in which we assume that *all events happened at the very last instant of
follow-up*. If this was true among the exposed, we would calculate person-time as
930 * 5 + 70 * 5 = 5,000 person-years and the incidence rate as 0.07 per 5 person-
years: numerically the same as the risk itself from Table 2.3. The incidence odds is
just the opposite: it is similar to an incidence rate in which all events occurred at
the very first instant of follow-up. Again, if this was true among the exposed, we
would calculate person time as 930 * 5 + 70 * 0 = 4,650 and an incidence rate of
0.075 per 5 person-years, identical to the odds in Table 2.3. You can work this out
for the unexposed subjects.

Thus, the incidence rate—which allows events to occur at various times during
follow-up rather than implicitly suggesting that all events occur at the end of
follow-up (as the risk) or the beginning of follow-up (as the odds)—is generally
expected to fall between the risk and the odds numerically when considered over
the same time period.[3]

---

3. Though, of course, the incidence rate has different units than the risk or the odds.

We can use the incidence rates in Table 2.5 to calculate the incidence rate difference as $0.725 - 0.0305 = 0.0421$ per 5 person-years. The incidence rate ratio is, similarly, $0.725/0.0305 = 2.38$ (and has no units). (For discussion of the relationship between Tables 2.3 and 2.5, see Box 2.2.)

2.2.7 Time Differences and Ratios

Consider the question of how some exposure (to compound C) might be associated with earlier menarche (onset of menses) in young women. Suppose further that, by age 18, 99% of individuals possessing XX chromosomes in the United States will have experienced menarche regardless of exposure. As such, long-term risk-type measures may be of limited or no utility: for example, risk difference by age 18 or even 16 is likely to be extremely small and uninformative. Contrasts in shorter term risks (e.g., the risk difference for the outcome of menarche by age 12) might be more useful, but these will ignore differences after the cutoff age. Incidence rate differences or ratios may be more useful here, but we also consider the difference (or ratio) in median times to event compared between two curves.

In Figure 2.1, we show two hypothetical curves for time until menarche in two groups: exposed (dotted line) and unexposed (solid black line). Here, we see that the exposure is associated with an earlier median age at menarche: median age in the exposed curve (where the "50%" line intersects with the dotted curve) is 12 years, while in the unexposed curve the median age is (similarly) 13 years. The difference in median age at menarche is therefore approximately 1 year. Note that the *time difference* (comparing exposed to unexposed) is $12 - 13 = -1$; the time ratio is $12/13 = 0.92$; this makes sense because the time to menarche is shorter

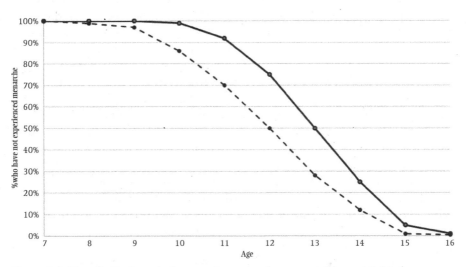

Figure 2.1 Hypothetical survival curves for menarche among girls aged 7–16, for an exposed group (*dotted line*) and unexposed group (*solid line*).
Data inspired by Freedman et al. (2002).

among the exposed girls (in the dotted curve). On the other hand, the risk at age 12 in the exposed (dotted curve) is 50%, calculated as 1 minus the proportion who have survived at this point (the survival proportion) of 50%. The risk in the unexposed (solid curve) is 25%, calculated as 1 minus the survival proportion of 75%. Thus, the risk difference of reaching menarche by age 12 is 50% − 25% = 25%. This makes sense as well because the proportion of girls who experience menarche by age 12 is higher in the exposed group than in the unexposed group. Notice that while the risk difference is positive (higher risk in the exposed) the time difference is negative (because higher risk means a generally shorter time to event in the exposed). This "flip" to the opposite side of the null for risk as compared with median time to event is a general (though not necessarily universal) rule. It is often perceived as counterintuitive, misunderstood, or forgotten, and indeed can be entirely missed if you calculate the survival difference [50% − 75%] rather than the risk difference [(1 − 50%) − (1 − 75%)] = [50% − 25%].

Now we consider how best to communicate to a parent concerned about the exposure in question. Putting aside questions of the individual applicability or generalizability of these findings, consider which of the following statements is clearer in communicating Figure 2.1:

1. The typical girl has a 25% higher risk of experiencing menarche by age 12 (on the absolute scale) if she is exposed compared to if she is unexposed.
2. The typical girl will experience menarche approximately 1 year earlier if she is exposed compared to if she is unexposed.

Both uses of "typical" are problematic—in the latter case, for example, most girls are not the median girl! Nonetheless, we would argue that the latter statement is clearer for communicating, especially to a nontechnical audience.

2.2.8 The Hazard Ratio

The hazard ratio is a measure of association used in time-to-event analysis. The hazard is defined as the "instantaneous rate"; that is, the rate at a given moment, conditional on not having yet experienced the event. The hazard ratio is then defined as the ratio between two hazards (e.g., the hazard among the exposed and among the unexposed). Despite wide usage, the hazard ratio is extremely difficult to interpret correctly, and the assumptions required to appropriately estimate hazard ratios are not well-understood. Even when well-understood these are frequently neither checked nor discussed. Further discussion of the hazard ratio is beyond our scope (see Hernán, 2010).

2.3 WHEN TO USE WHICH MEASURES OF ASSOCIATION

In this text, we will concentrate largely on difference measures (in particular, the risk difference) and ratio measures (in particular, the risk ratio).

It is widely agreed that public health questions—questions of the form, "What intervention should we take in this population?"—are best answered using absolute measures, such as the risk difference (Poole, 2010). This is because public health is ultimately about helping people—and often about the cost-effectiveness of a particular intervention, a key component of which is the number of people helped. For example, how many heart attacks would we prevent if all participants were to quit smoking? How many deaths would we prevent over 10 years if all participants cut all animal products from their diets?

In contrast, the risk ratio does not tell us how many people will be affected or the absolute scale of the risks. A risk ratio of 2 might represent the comparison of 2 in 1,000 to 1 in 1,000 (a risk difference of 0.1%, or one person in a thousand), or of 2 in 10 to 1 in 10 (a risk difference of 10%, or one in ten). Clearly there are potentially substantial implications in comparing differences of 1 in 1,000 and 1 in 10 (e.g., with respect to implementation efficiency for comparable interventions), but the risk ratio obscures this difference. Thus, one should prefer the risk difference (and absolute measures more broadly) for communicating the public health importance of measures.

What use, then, is the risk ratio (or ratio measures in general)? Opinions differ, but it is argued that, as a tool for talking about how individual risks may change, a statement like "given that you seem like one of the people we studied, we expect you have double the risk" may be more meaningful to many individuals than a statement like "we expect your risk to be higher by 5 parts in 100"—especially if the baseline levels of risk are well-understood.[4] Thus, ratio measures may be useful for communicating to individuals and in helping individuals make choices about their health. However, there are clearly situations in which a risk difference is superior for this purpose as well. There are also situations in which ratio measures are used to scare rather than inform. Finally, we reiterate that, on the ratio scale, the risk ratio is preferable to the odds ratio, recognizing again that we sometimes estimate an odds ratio for data, design, or statistical reasons—and that when the risks are low, the odds ratio will give us much the same qualitative picture as the risk ratio.

2.4 SUMMARY

In this chapter, we discussed several measures of association, on both the absolute and relative scales, which are central to epidemiologic research. Key measures include risk differences, risk ratios, odds ratios, incidence rates and differences, and time differences and ratios. We started to discuss interpretations of each measure, the null values of each, and relative advantages and disadvantages.

---

4. Which is a very good reason to always report the estimated risk in the unexposed group or overall population alongside the risk ratio. Such information allows the person interpreting the finding some perspective about what that number really means.

In Chapter 3, we will discuss (among other things) the circumstances under which such measures can be interpreted as estimates of causal effects; in future chapters, we will discuss study designs and approaches to estimating both associations and causal effects.

REFERENCES

Freedman, D. S., Khan, L. K., Serdula, M. K., Dietz, W. H., Srinivasan, S. R., & Berenson, G. S. (2002). Relation of age at menarche to race, time period, and anthropometric dimensions: The Bogalusa Heart Study. *Pediatrics, 110*(4), e43.

Hernán, M. A. (2010). The hazards of hazard ratios. *Epidemiology, 21*(1), 13–15.

Poole, C. (2010). On the origin of risk relativism. *Epidemiology, 21*(1), 3–9.

3

Causal Inference, Causal Effect Estimation, and Systematic Error

There is a rich and growing literature on causal inference and causal effect estimation (Greenland, 2017; Hernán & Robins, 2019). Here, our goal is a brief introduction to concepts, terms, and notation. Many concepts introduced here will be developed further in subsequent chapters. For example, we introduce the idea of confounding in this chapter, but expand on that concept in discussing randomized trials (in Chapter 5) and observational cohort studies (Chapter 6).

In this chapter, we discuss elements of causal inference, causal effect estimation, systematic error, and related concepts. Along the way, we will discuss the circumstances under which we can interpret the measures of association discussed in the previous chapter and estimates of those measures, as measures and estimates of causal effects. As noted in the Acknowledgements, this Chapter in particular owes a particular debt of intellectual influence to numerous key scientists cited below. Hopefully, the citations throughout the Chapter reflect this debt; if not, however, I want to be clear that in this Chapter more than others I am standing on the shoulders of numerous others.

3.1 EPIDEMIOLOGIC PARADIGMS: DESCRIPTIVE, PREDICTIVE, CAUSAL

Epidemiology is the core science of public health, and public health is the field dedicated to intervening to improve health at the population level. Of course, we only want to intervene on factors which are causal: to intervene on noncausal exposures will not change health (or, at least, not in the way we think). For example: drinking alcohol can increase risk of car accidents, while drinking coffee generally does not. But if it was true that people who drink alcohol are more likely than others to drink coffee, we might observe an association between drinking coffee and increased risk of car accidents—an association actually due to the association of alcohol with both coffee consumption and risk of car accidents. An observed association between coffee consumption and risk of car accidents may help us *predict* who is likely to be in a car accident (coffee drinkers); but, in this

Epidemiology by Design: A Causal Approach to the Health Sciences. Daniel Westreich, Oxford University Press (2020). © Oxford University Press.
DOI: 10.1093/oso/9780190665760.001.0001

case, using that information as a reason to persuade people to stop drinking coffee (i.e., to intervene on coffee consumption) in an effort to prevent car accidents is clearly misguided because there is no causal effect of coffee on accident risk.

A chief concern of epidemiology, therefore, is estimating *causal effects*: understanding the impact of exposure to some factor or treatment on health outcomes. However, there are two other epidemiologic paradigms which we will address in this book: descriptive and predictive epidemiology. Both of these are addressed in more depth in Chapter 4, but we discuss them briefly here because doing so helps delineate what is meant by causal epidemiology. *Descriptive epidemiology* is concerned with communicating the observed world as it is—for example, in characterizing the prevalence of some disease in the population. Whereas *predictive epidemiology* is concerned with diagnostic testing (given your characteristics or test results, are you likely to have a particular disease which is not directly observable?) and prognostics (given your characteristics, are you likely to acquire a particular disease? Given your characteristics and your disease, how will your health evolve in the next months or years?). The borders of these paradigms are fuzzy, of course: diagnostic testing can be seen as a form of description of the world.

The borders of these paradigms are fuzzy, of course: for example, diagnostic testing can be seen as a form of description of the world. Both descriptive and predictive epidemiology are important to public health: descriptive epidemiology, often in the form of disease surveillance efforts (Chapter 4), tells us how prevalent a particular disease might be and thus helps us prioritize resources. Predictive epidemiology may help patients understand whether they have a disease or how their disease may progress over time (arguably the domain of clinical epidemiology), but it may also help inform prevention efforts by forecasting future disease burden. Again, we go into more depth on both these paradigms in the next chapter: here, we concern ourselves chiefly with identification and estimation of causal effects.

3.2 COUNTERFACTUAL THINKING AND POTENTIAL OUTCOMES

Consider Jimmy, who is driving his car on the freeway. Jimmy gets a text message, so he picks up his phone to read it and he nearly immediately gets into an accident. We might reasonably ask, "Did reading the text message cause Jimmy's accident?" But what is it that we mean—really mean—when we ask this question?

What we mean is often something like the following: "What if Jimmy had *not* read the text message: would he, nonetheless, still have gotten into the accident?" When we ask that question, we just as often have in our heads this set of responses:

> If Jimmy would *still* have gotten into the accident *even if he had not read the text message*, then reading the text message did *not* cause his accident.
>
> But if Jimmy would *not* have gotten into the accident had he *not* read the text message, then reading that text message *did* cause his accident.

That what-if question, a kind of experiment we run in our own head, captures the essence of a *counterfactual* approach to causality. We compare what factually happened (Jimmy read the text and got into a car accident) with what would have happened if, counter to fact, had Jimmy not read the text. This approach—sometimes called "but-for" (or *sine qua non*) causality in the law—is closely related to *potential outcomes*, words which are often used synonymously with counterfactuals.

To help us think clearly through these ideas, we introduce some simple notation. We consider a two-category exposure X, for example "current smoking" compared with "no current smoking." Alternatively, we can think of X as a treatment chosen by a patient or assigned in a randomized trial, such as "assigned to receive an influenza immunization" compared with "assigned to receive a placebo injection." In general we will consider $X = 1$ to indicate the "exposed" or "treated" category (e.g., exposed to current smoking or assignment to immunization) and $X = 0$ to indicate "unexposed" or "untreated."

We consider also a two-category outcome Y, such as "had a heart attack within 1 year" compared with "did not have a heart attack within 1 year" or "was hospitalized within 30 days" compared with "was not hospitalized within 30 days" or "died within 10 years" compared with "alive at the end of 10 years." In general we will consider $Y = 1$ to indicate "had a poor health outcome" (e.g., had a heart attack within 1 year) and $Y = 0$ to indicate "did not have a poor health outcome" (e.g., did not have a heart attack within 1 year). Both X and Y are specific to individuals, so both may be subscripted with i to indicate which individual is being considered: i can range from 1 to n or 1 to N, where n (N) is often used to indicate the number of individuals in the study (population).

As in previous chapters, we make several simplifying assumptions about risks and related measures. In particular, we assume that the time period over which study participants were followed is fixed and follow-up is complete (no one disappears, such that we do not record their outcome status). We also assume no *competing risks*, that no other events occurred which prevent the outcome of interest from occurring: for example, we assume that hospitalization within 30 days was not prevented by a study participant's death. In some cases we will leave the time period in which the outcome must have occurred implicit, although it is generally necessary to state it (see Chapters 1 and 2). Such assumptions are not necessary and can be relaxed under some circumstances.

3.2.1 An Example

Now consider an experiment in which we flip a coin to determine the treatment (say, an active drug or a placebo) to which an individual is assigned. In particular, suppose we wish to randomize individuals who have just suffered a first heart attack to receive either a single dose of a new, long-acting drug or a single dose of a placebo; we will then follow all individuals for a year to assess the risk of death in each treatment group. Consider one participant in this randomized trial, Sarah, who adheres to the treatment to which she is assigned in the trial.

Before we flip the coin to assign Sarah to one arm of the trial or another, Sarah has two *potential outcomes*. There is her potential outcome under assignment to exposure $X = 1$: the outcome Sarah would experience if the coin comes up heads and she is assigned to receive the active drug. And there is her potential outcome under assignment to exposure $X = 0$: the outcome Sarah would experience if the coin comes up tails and she is assigned to receive the placebo.[1] We designate these potential outcomes $Y^{x=1}$ and $Y^{x=0}$, respectively. Both of these potential outcomes are mathematical abstractions; we may get to observe the value of one of these potential outcomes in reality, but not more than one. Potential outcomes were first described by Neyman in 1923 (1923/1990) and then popularized by Rubin in 1974 and thereafter.

Sarah has two potential outcomes—and each potential outcome has two possible values: at the end of the year of follow-up, she might be alive or dead. Specifically, if she is assigned the active drug, then, by the end of the year, she may have died ($Y^{x=1} = 1$) or not died ($Y^{x=1} = 0$); likewise, if she is assigned the placebo, by the end of the year she may have died ($Y^{x=0} = 1$) or not died ($Y^{x=0} = 0$). Note that in the case of an exposure (or treatment) with more than two categories, or which is continuous, there are more than two potential outcomes for each individual. If the outcome is continuous, there are more than two possible outcome values.

After we flip the coin, Sarah is assigned to one of the two possible treatments: active drug or placebo. Suppose the coin comes up heads, and so Sarah's exposure is set to $X = 1$. We then follow Sarah for a year and measure her actual outcome. At this point, we can safely assume that her *factual* outcome is equal to her potential outcome under $X = 1$, specifically $Y^{x=1}$. Her potential outcome under $X = 0$, however, will never and can never be known: $Y^{x=0}$ has become *counterfactual*— indeed, it became counterfactual at the moment of treatment assignment. While Sarah's potential outcome under $X = 1$ has become factual, her potential outcome under $X = 0$ remains *counter to fact*: she was not (in fact) assigned to $X = 0$, and so $Y^{x=0}$ remains unknown. This illustrates a subtle difference in usage between potential outcomes and counterfactuals. Again, numerous investigators use these terms interchangeably, typically without introducing confusion.

3.2.2 Individual Causal Effects

Now that we have introduced the preceding notation and ideas, we can define the *individual causal effect* of X for Sarah as the difference between (i) her potential outcome under assignment to $X = 1$ and (ii) her potential outcome under assignment to $X = 0$, or $Y^{x=1} - Y^{x=0}$. In Sarah's case, suppose that, after assignment to the active drug, we discover that her outcome under that exposure was to live (i.e., that $Y^{x=1} = 0$); and suppose we also know that had she been assigned to the placebo she would have died (i.e., that $Y^{x=0} = 1$). Then her individual causal effect is $Y^{x=1} - Y^{x=0} = 0 - 1 = -1$: the causal effect of treatment in Sarah is -1, the negative

---

1. Note that here X refers to Sarah's treatment *assignment*, which is not necessarily the same as actually taking the treatment. Unless Sarah is perfectly adherent to her treatment assignment, the potential outcomes for treatment assignment can differ from the potential outcomes for actually taking the treatment.

sign indicating that taking the active drug will *prevent* (rather than cause) the death she would have suffered had she (counter-to-fact) taken the placebo.

We have now defined an individual causal effect, but there is a problem with this definition. One of the two components in Sarah's causal effect ($Y^{x=0}$) was counterfactual, and what is counterfactual was not observed in reality. Which means that—except in made-up data—Sarah's *individual causal effect can never be known for sure*. We can guess at an individual causal effect under strong assumptions—with our previous example of Jimmy who checked his text messages at an inopportune time, many people would feel comfortable betting on the idea that checking his text messages caused his accident. But we cannot know for sure because at least one component of every individual causal effect is counterfactual and thus missing. It is for this reason that it is sometimes said that the "fundamental problem of causal inference" is missing data (Holland, 1986).

3.2.3 Average Causal Effects

We cannot (in general) assess individual causal effects, but we can assess *average causal effects* under additional conditions (see the later discussion in the section "Causal Identification Conditions"). Average causal effects (or population average causal effects) are the average differences in outcomes comparing two treatments or exposures at the population level.

Continuing with our example of a trial of a new long-acting drug versus placebo to prevent death within 1 year: like Sarah, each person in that study population has two potential outcomes, one under each treatment assignment, and each potential outcome could take on one of two possible values, alive or dead at the end of 1 year. In the whole population of N people, we can describe the number of people with each combination of potential outcomes and values in a 2×2 table, as shown in Table 3.1.

In Table 3.1, A counts the number of people for whom the potential outcomes under both $X = 0$ and $X = 1$ are equal to 1: these are people who will get the outcome ($Y = 1$) regardless of treatment ($X = 1$ or $X = 0$). Since the outcome is bad, we sometimes designate these individuals "doomed" to get the outcome (see Box 3.1). Who might such people be? Consider a person who dies in a car accident a week after the trial begins and so is counted as an outcome in this trial: it is reasonable to assume that the car accident would have occurred and the individual would have died regardless of whether that person had received active drug or placebo. Similarly, D counts the number of people for whom both potential outcomes are

Table 3.1 A 2 × 2 TABLE OF POTENTIAL OUTCOME TYPES

	$Y^{x=1} = 1$	$Y^{x=1} = 0$	Total
$Y^{x=0} = 1$	A	B	$A + B$
$Y^{x=0} = 0$	C	D	$C + D$
Total	$A + C$	$B + D$	$A + B + C + D = N$

Box 3.1

Are Potential Outcomes Predetermined?

Throughout this chapter, we discuss people who are certain "causal types"—who are doomed or immune. This nomenclature assumes that potential outcomes are predetermined: it might be that a person gets a disease or escapes it, or only gets it if exposed (or not exposed)—we do not know which. But we assume that each person has an *intrinsic response type*, and it is this response type which dictates what her outcomes are under each exposure condition. While this assumption is helpful in building our understanding, it may well not be true: potential outcomes may be stochastic—that is, random rather than predetermined (VanderWeele & Robins, 2012). However, the assumption of determinism is helpful in clarifying causal thinking.

---

equal to 0: these people are "immune" from experiencing the outcome because no matter the exposure they will not experience the outcome. *B* represents the number of people who will experience the outcome when unexposed but *not* when exposed and so those who are "protected" from the harmful outcome by their exposure, and *C* represents the number of people who experience the outcome only when exposed and are therefore "harmed" by their exposure.

In Table 3.1, an average causal effect could be calculated as the difference between (i) the proportion of people in the entire population who would experience the outcome under exposure ($X = 1$), which is $(A + C)/(A + B + C + D)$, and (ii) the proportion of people in the same population who would experience the outcome under non-exposure ($X = 0$), which is $(A + B)/(A + B + C + D)$. Using this information, we can calculate the *average causal risk difference* as:

$$\frac{A+C}{A+B+C+D} - \frac{A+B}{A+B+C+D}$$

which can be rewritten in terms of probability (Pr) of the outcomes as

$$\Pr\left(Y^{x=1} = 1\right) - \Pr\left(Y^{x=0} = 1\right)$$

or more simply as

$$\Pr\left(Y^{1}\right) - \Pr\left(Y^{0}\right).$$

This is, simply, the difference between the risk of the outcome if everyone in the population were assigned $X = 1$ and the risk of the outcome if everyone in the population were assigned $X = 0$. We could further generalize this measure by expressing it in terms of expectations rather than probabilities (i.e., $E(Y^1) - E(Y^0)$), which is a difference measure for any Y, including continuous-valued health outcomes such as weight or forced expiratory volume in 1 second.

The average causal risk ratio can likewise be written as

$$\frac{\Pr(Y^{x=1} = 1)}{\Pr(Y^{x=0} = 1)} = \frac{\Pr(Y^1)}{\Pr(Y^0)}.$$

This 2×2 table of potential outcomes was built out of individual data—an individual's assignment to group A, B, C, or D depends on information about the joint distribution of their potential outcomes, which we have already noted is unavailable to us. Recall that, in Chapter 2, we discussed how to estimate a risk difference and risk ratio from observed data. In the next section, we address some conditions under which we can interpret such measures of association, estimated from real data, as estimates of causal effects.

3.3 CAUSAL IDENTIFICATION CONDITIONS

As noted earlier, we cannot identify all potential outcomes because, at most, only one potential outcome will ever be factually realized. However, we can assess causal effects in real data if we assume (hopefully with good reason) that we have met several causal identification conditions. Specifically, then, our goal is to understand what it takes to interpret an associational risk difference (or risk ratio, etc.) such as

$$\Pr(Y = 1 \mid X = 1) - \Pr(Y = 1 \mid X = 0),$$

as an average causal risk difference,

$$\Pr(Y^{x=1} = 1) - \Pr(Y^{x=0} = 1).$$

The causal identification conditions have received extensive treatments elsewhere (Greenland, 2017; Hernán & Robins, 2019). Here, we go over four key conditions which together are *sufficient* for identification of causal effects in real data. That is, when all four conditions are met, we can be reasonably assured that our measured association estimates the causal effect of interest. The key conditions we describe here are *temporality, causal consistency, exchangeability*, and *no measurement error*. We will also discuss *conditional exchangeability with positivity* as a substitute for the simpler *exchangeability*.

Again, we emphasize that this set of conditions is sufficient; it is not necessary for all causal effect estimation. There are other sufficient sets of conditions as well, such as those used for *instrumental variables* (see Chapter 8). In the Appendix to this chapter, we show how these four causal identification conditions help us make a causal interpretation from an association (i.e., considering the two equations immediately above, how we move from the first equation to the second). Before we discuss these conditions, however, we must address an additional, vital condition, or assumption, in the estimation of causal effects: identification of the target population.

3.3.1 Target Populations and Study Samples

Again, our goal here is causal effect estimation from data. But, thus far in this chapter, we have not considered *in which population* we want to estimate the causal effect. The *target population* is "the group of people about which our scientific or public-health question asks, and therefore for which we want to estimate the causal effect of an exposure," according to Maldonado and Greenland (2002). This group is also frequently described as a *source* or *base population* (Porta, 2014).[2] When we do not explicitly discuss a target, or source, population, it may seem reasonable to assume that the target population is the data we are analyzing, which we call the *study sample*. In the real world, this is very often not true.

Briefly, consider a study of 1,000 people of how a new drug agent treats a disease compared to a placebo. The goal of such a study is almost never to estimate a causal effect which only applies to those 1,000 people. Rather, the goal (quite often) is to obtain information that applies to all those individuals who might be eligible to use the new drug agent under study. Likewise, we might perform a study in North Carolina, but want to know how those results apply to an external target population (people in South Carolina). We will discuss target populations further in Chapter 5 and Chapter 9. For the remainder of this chapter we assume that our target population is exactly the data in front of us, that is that we wish to estimate causal effects only in our study sample.

3.3.2 Causal Identification Conditions

Now, we discuss the causal identification conditions. It is unlikely that these causal identification conditions will be fully transparent to you the first time they are encountered: repeated exposure—to this chapter, to other sources (Hernán & Robins, 2019), and also to the way in which these concepts arise again in subsequent chapters on the study designs—is the surest route to increased understanding. So, don't worry if the causal identification conditions are not entirely clear the first time you read them.

---

2. A key difference in usage, however, is that "source population" carries with it the implication that this is the source of the data in your study. However, this may not be the case: we may wish to apply the results of the study to an entirely external population as well. Both cases together are more generally covered by the phrase "target population."

3.3.3 Temporality

Temporality is the condition that things which are causes precede their purported effects in time. If we wish to assess the effect of aspirin use on risk of heart attack, we must be sure that study participants' use of aspirin occurred prior to time of heart attack. Temporality might be violated when (for example) a study subject already has the outcome at the time of exposure—for example, a participant has incipient liver cancer at the start of a randomized trial in which the outcome is liver cancer. *Reverse causality* is a particular manifestation of this phenomenon in which the (undiagnosed) existence of the outcome affects an individual's exposure status; for example, in a study of the effect of smoking on lung disease (e.g., chronic obstructive pulmonary disease [COPD]), this might occur if early symptoms of as-yet-undiagnosed COPD lead an individual to stop smoking.

3.3.4 Causal Consistency

Causal consistency, or sometimes simply *consistency*, is the idea that *among people who were exposed*, their outcome was no different than it would have been if they had been assigned that exposure—and the same is true for the unexposed. This idea is key in interpreting the observed outcomes as the potential outcomes: in the chapter Appendix, we show how the application of causal consistency allows us to move one step from an association to an estimate of causal effect (Hernán & Robins, 2019).

When can we assume that this condition is true? One crucial aspect of consistency relates to the question of whether there is meaningful variation in the observed exposure or treatment. Suppose we want to know the effect of daily aspirin on risk of heart attack. For the exposure of "take aspirin daily," we may view dose of aspirin (e.g., 81 mg vs. 162 mg) as meaningful variation in the exposure in that we could imagine a substantially different causal effect for each dose. At the same time, we might view the issue of whether the aspirin is taken in the early morning versus late at night as irrelevant; however, if we discovered that the physiologic effects of aspirin differed substantially by whether you went to sleep immediately after taking the aspirin or not, then the latter variation would be considered meaningful. Consistency, then, is in part the assumption that any variations in the treatment or exposure being studied are irrelevant to the causal mechanism being studied: an idea often summarized as *treatment variation irrelevance.*

Questions of treatment variation irrelevance—of what constitutes a "meaningful" variation in treatment—is decided on a per-study, per-exposure basis, often after discussion among experts in the field. That said, this can become a particular issue when considering health-relevant demographic attributes such as race, sex, gender, or socioeconomic status. While strong arguments can (and have!) been made that all of these complex factors can be regarded as causes of disease, what precisely "cause" means is difficult because each of these words can mean various things depending on both speaker and context. For example, investigators often explore biological sex as a "cause" when they are in fact more interested in effects due to gender or discrimination based on gender presentation (which is not the same as sex), or due to hormone levels (which vary with sex but also with numerous other factors).

Likewise, numerous studies in the literature examine differences in health outcomes by self-reported racial identity and then attribute part or all those differences to genetic differences between the races. However, genetic differences between races are extremely minor, and it is almost never the case that we can reliably attribute observed differences in health status to such minor genetic differences (Cooper, 2013; Kaufman, Cooper, & McGee, 1997).

One particular aspect of treatment variation worth calling out is *interference*, also called *dependent happenings* or *spillover effects*. Interference is a situation in which *my* exposure has an effect on *your* potential outcome. Interference may be most easily understood in an infectious diseases setting: consider a treatment of an influenza vaccine. If I am exposed to the influenza vaccine, this can easily have an effect on my daughter's risk of acquiring influenza *independent of my daughter's vaccine status*. This is because my being immunized may decrease her exposure to and thus risk of acquiring influenza. Indeed, the idea of *herd immunity*—that when sufficient numbers of people are vaccinated against a disease in a population, the nonvaccinated members of that population will be protected as well—is based precisely on the existence of interference effects of this type. We can therefore expect the observed effects of this vaccine in a population to vary with the vaccine status of those around them: a form of treatment variation which seems highly relevant. While interference is a serious consideration when it arises, we frequently assume no interference as part of our consistency assumption and in noninfectious diseases settings this is often a reasonable assumption. However, there may be considerable spillover effects in infectious diseases settings, as well as with certain social phenomena.

There is at least one other use of the word "consistency" worth mentioning in this context. In statistics and biostatistics, a *consistent* estimator of a particular quantity is one which converges to the true value of that quantity as the number of data points increases: this is distinct from causal consistency. Somewhat related, "no interference" is considered by some investigators to be equivalent to or a subset of the *stable unit treatment value assumption* (SUTVA; see Hernán & Robins, 2019, for a discussion). For discussion of the relation of consistency to the notion of "well-defined interventions" see Box 3.2.

3.3.5 Exchangeability

Exchangeability is *informally* the condition that study participants who are exposed (or treated) have the same average pre-exposure (or pre-treatment) risk of the outcome as study participants who are unexposed (or untreated). Here, pre-exposure (pre-treatment) means "aside from any risk conferred by the exposure (treatment) itself." An alternate formulation of the same idea is that, if there were no causal effect of the treatment on anyone in the study, would the treated

Box 3.2

WELL-DEFINED INTERVENTIONS

One ongoing debate in the causal inference literature is whether we must have a "well-defined intervention" or "realistic intervention" in order to identify a causal effect. This seems obviously not to be the case, in part because "well-defined" is itself not always well-defined and in part because what is not realistic today may be entirely realistic in 10 years. For example, it seems uncontroversial that single-nucleotide polymorphisms (SNPs) can have a causal effect on health outcomes; this is true even though—at the time of this writing, though this may soon change—we have no means of intervening to correct or change such genetic issues.

The perspective of this textbook is, first, that having a well-defined intervention in mind can help clarify questions of consistency. And, second, that it is perfectly reasonable to estimate causal effects when a realistic intervention does not exist: SNPs being a useful case in point. However, it is clearly the case that there is no immediate public health application of an estimated causal effect of something we cannot change. Such an estimate may still be useful, of course: such an estimate might spur the development of interventions against the exposure. Indeed, vaccine development programs sometimes emerge from estimates of the causal effect of the disease agent that they target.

Nonetheless, when confronted with a causal hypothesis concerning an exposure for which no intervention currently exists, it can be clarifying to ask why the question is being asked and whether there is a more useful question that might be asked instead. For example, although sex chromosomes are a cause of certain health outcomes, we have no intervention to change them. So sometimes, at least, we might be better off asking questions about downstream effects of sex chromosomes that we might be able to change: for example, the experience of sex and gender discrimination at the individual and systemic levels. While the latter is difficult to change, one can at least imagine a pathway to changing experiences of sexism, whereas the idea of changing chromosomes seems far more difficult (both biologically and ethically).

In passing, we will note that a useful "trick" for clarifying a research question is to ask: If I could design a randomized trial for this exposure, what would that randomized trial be? Who would be included? What treatments would participants be randomized to? Such an exercise, as we discuss later, can be clarifying, in part because it forces a clear articulation of a treatment—which can then inform analysis of less ideal data.

and untreated groups have the same average risk of the outcome? For example, in a study of the impact of a new drug on the outcome of heart attack, 40-year-olds would not (broadly speaking) be considered exchangeable with 60-year-olds because risk of heart attack increases with age—quite aside from the effects of the drug under study. Another informal way to state this condition is that if exchangeability holds, then the risk of the exposed can stand in for the risk of the unexposed if—counter to fact—the unexposed had been exposed; and, similarly, the risk of the unexposed can stand in for the risk of the exposed if—counter to fact—the exposed had been unexposed.

Formally, the issue of exchangeability is about the statistical independence between the potential outcomes and the exposure or treatment actually received by participants in a study, which is typically stated as $Y^x \amalg X$ for all values of x. For dichotomous Y and X this can also be written as $\Pr\left(Y^x \mid X = 1\right) = \Pr(Y^x \mid X = 0)$, which states that the risk of Y for a set level of X (specifically, x) is the same among those observed to be treated and those observed to be untreated (Hernán & Robins, 2019). In the chapter Appendix, we show how the application of exchangeability, as with causal consistency, allows us to take an additional step from an association to an estimate of causal effect.

When does exchangeability hold, or not hold? While we will discuss this issue at more length in the later section on systematic error and in subsequent chapters, it is clear that, in a large population, random assignment of treatment (e.g., flipping a coin to decide who receives treatment and who does not) will on average produce exchangeable samples. This is because over the long run, for every 60-year-old who is treated there will be a 60-year-old who is not, and, likewise, for every 40-year-old who is treated there will be a 40-year-old who is not treated. So, on average, the proportions of 40- and 60-year-olds will be the same in the two groups, and so—aside from any effect of the treatment itself—the average risk of the outcome will be the same in the two groups as well. Lack of exchangeability, on the other hand, is generally due to the systematic errors *confounding* and *selection bias* and is often what people mean when they repeat the statement that "correlation is not causation"—although we are quick to remind you that *correlation is not not-causation*, as well. These systematic errors are discussed in greater depth later.

Again, we are satisfied that the exchangeability assumption is met sufficiently to estimate an average causal effect if pre-treatment risks (i.e., the potential outcomes in absence of exposure) in our two comparison groups are the same on average. Note that individual causal effects—though we cannot estimate them—would likewise meet the exchangeability condition as well, in that any individual at a particular moment in time has the same baseline risk of an outcome whether they are treated or untreated immediately thereafter.

3.3.6 Conditional Exchangeability

In observational studies, the reasons that individuals wind up exposed (either by choice or by circumstance) frequently involve exactly those factors which also affect the affect risk of the outcome. Thus, in observational settings, the average pre-exposure risk among those who are exposed is *not* (in general) the same as the average pre-exposure risk among those who are not exposed. For example, as earlier, if 40-year-olds are more likely to start smoking than 60-year-olds, then the smokers are not exchangeable with the nonsmokers (and we would say that the effects of smoking are "confounded by age," see later discussion). Here, when average pre-treatment risk of the outcome is *not* the same across exposure groups, we must try to deal analytically with variables like age. If we can meet exchangeability after accounting for (conditioning on) additional variables such as age, we call this *conditional exchangeability*. The formal statement of conditional exchangeability is only slightly different from the formal statement of exchangeability noted earlier: specifically, $Y^x \perp\!\!\!\perp X \mid Z$ for all values of x, where Z is all relevant covariates (in our example in this paragraph, age; see Hernán & Robins, 2019).

To explain further: recall from above that exchangeability implies that *the risk of the exposed can stand in for the risk of the unexposed, if—counter to fact—the unexposed had been exposed (and vice versa)*. Conditional exchangeability says similarly that *the risk of the exposed can stand in for the risk of the unexposed*, conditional on certain additional variables, *if—counter to fact—the unexposed had been exposed (and vice versa)*. Back to our populations of 40-year-olds and 60-year-olds, it might be that the risk of exposed 40-year-olds can stand in for the risk of unexposed 40-year-olds, had those unexposed 40-year-olds in fact been exposed and, likewise, that the risk of exposed 60-year-olds can stand in for the risk of unexposed 60-year-olds had those unexposed 60-year-olds in fact been exposed and so on. The identification and choice of variables for conditional exchangeability based on causal diagrams will be explained later, in Section 3.4 on causal diagrams and confounding.

3.3.7 Positivity

But what if there were no exposed 60-year-olds in our study—if the only exposed people were 40-year-olds? Conditional exchangeability introduces new variables to our system, and the need to deal with other variables introduces another condition to be met, namely *positivity*. Informally, positivity is the condition that all subjects must have a non-zero chance of receiving either treatment under study: in this case, 40-year-olds must have a nonzero chance of both initiating and not initiating smoking, and the same must be true for 60-year-olds. Positivity is about the *relationship of the exposure to the variables required for conditional exchangeability*—thus, once we have chosen the set of variables necessary for conditional exchangeability, the outcome is no longer part of the discussion of positivity. The close linkage between these two conditions sometimes leads us to refer to them jointly as *conditional exchangeability with positivity*.

The formal statement of positivity condition is $\Pr(X = x \mid Z = z) > 0$, where Z is all covariates used for conditional exchangeability, and z is all combinations of those covariates present in the data under study (Hernán & Robins, 2019). Thus, there must be a greater than zero probability of *any treatment or exposure condition* for all observed combinations of the covariates relevant to conditional exchangeability.

Broadly, there are two essential ways in which we might lack positivity: structural (or deterministic) and stochastic. In *structural nonpositivity*, there is a segment of the population under study which has no opportunity for exposure for structural (e.g., physical) reasons: if we are asking about the effect of hysterectomy on some later health outcome, then study subjects who lack a uterus cannot experience the exposure. In this case, the best course is likely to exclude such subjects from an estimate of causal effect—there is no reason to ask the question of the impact of a hysterectomy in these subjects in the first place. *Stochastic nonpositivity* is a data, rather than structural, phenomenon. For example, we might have a population in which by chance no one under the age of 50 is a smoker, and everyone over the age of 50 is a nonsmoker. While there is no physiologic barrier to being a smoker under age 50, in such a population it becomes difficult (though not impossible) to separate effects of smoking and age.

3.3.8 No Measurement Error

No measurement error is *not* broadly discussed as a causal identification condition, but it is worth noting here (and it is useful in the chapter Appendix as well). If the exposure or outcome (or covariates required for conditional exchangeability) is measured with error, we sometimes cannot estimate a valid causal effect even under otherwise ideal conditions—for example, a perfectly conducted randomized trial that ensured temporality, unconditional exchangeability, and consistency (see Chapter 5). We therefore regard lack of measurement error as a helpful condition for causal effect estimation, although there are rare cases when measurement error can actually be helpful (see quasi-experiments in Chapter 6). We add briefly that one can view treatment variation irrelevance (consistency) as an issue of measurement error. If the exposure is defined as "takes any amount of aspirin daily," then both 81 mg and 162 mg doses of aspirin are valid. But if the exposure of interest is really "one 81 mg aspirin daily," then the classification of 162 mg of daily aspirin as "exposed" is in fact *misclassification*, a type of measurement error.

3.3.9 Summary

The preceding conditions—temporality, consistency (primarily treatment variation irrelevance, including no interference), exchangeability (or alternatively conditional exchangeability with positivity), and no measurement error—are useful, though not strictly necessary (Greenland, 2017), for nonparametric identification of causal effects from data.[3] Practical considerations, such as the "curse of dimensionality," often force us to make additional assumptions encoded in statistical models to estimate effects. The chief such assumption is that such models

---

3. "Nonparametric" is a term which here means approximately "model-free" or "without using a regression model" or "directly from data."

are correctly specified (Keil et al., 2018). Machine learning approaches can help us ensure correct model specification with far fewer assumptions, though they may introduce additional statistical issues (Naimi & Balzer, 2018; van der Laan & Rose, 2011).

When treatment is randomized, it is often reasonable to assume that many or all of these conditions are met, for reasons we will discuss in Chapter 5. In such a setting, one can usually estimate causal effects for the study sample from a pair of survival curves or a simple 2 × 2 table and be reasonably confident in the validity of those estimates. However, when treatment is *not* randomized, we often do not know whether we have met these conditions—perhaps most centrally whether we have met conditional exchangeability. In such settings, if we wish to interpret measures of association estimated from data as causal effect estimates, we must assume that these conditions hold: in this case, we would assume that we have conditional exchangeability given certain variables. One way to be transparent about such assumptions is to encode some of them in a diagram of your hypothesized causal system.

3.4 CAUSAL DIAGRAMS

Causal diagrams were introduced into mainstream epidemiologic literature in 1999, in a paper by Greenland, Pearl, and Robins (1999) and are a useful tool for thinking through questions of systematic error in a study, particularly questions of (conditional) exchangeability. Here, we concentrate on a particular type of causal diagram called *causal directed acyclic graphs* (alternatively, DAGs or causal DAGs), although *single-world intervention graphs* (SWIGs) are also a useful technology for causal effect estimation and additionally map more directly onto potential outcomes than do causal DAGs. In this section we introduce DAGs and explain briefly how to use them to identify conditional exchangeability.

DAGs are simply a collection of nodes (representing variables) and single-headed arrows connecting those nodes (*directed* arrows connecting nodes into a *graph*), where there are no *cycles* of arrows (you cannot start at a node, follow arrows, and return to the same node). Arrows indicate causal relationships: an arrow from X to Y indicates that X is a cause of Y (and therefore that changing X may change Y). DAGs explicitly forbid double-headed arrows.[4]

For example, if we wish to know the effect of X on Y, we would start by drawing a node labeled X, a node labeled Y, and a single-headed arrow from X to Y indicating the possibility of a causal effect of X on Y (specifically, the possibility that intervening to change X will result in a change in Y; Figure 3.1, left). In most cases, we understand the nodes X and Y to be random variables representing

---

4. Although some investigators informally use no-headed arrows in a DAG to indicate a non-causal association between two variables. Such no-headed arrows make the structure formally improper, and so it might be clearer to create an additional variable which affects both of the two variables.

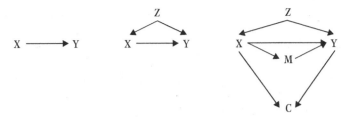

Figure 3.1 Three causal directed acyclic graphs of increasing complexity.

values taken on by an individual; thus X and Y in Figure 3.1 could both have an i subscript indicating that they are individual variables. However, such a subscript is typically omitted.

From this base, we create other nodes for other variables we believe to be relevant to the $X{\rightarrow}Y$ relationship (see Box 3.3): for example, we could include a joint cause of both X and Y and call it Z. We draw a node for Z and then draw single-headed arrows from Z to X (Z is a cause of X) and from Z to Y (Z is a cause of Y) (Figure 3.1, center). We might expand that figure to include an additional possible pathway between X and Y that includes a new variable, M, and finally add in the idea that X and Y both affect (i.e., cause) some additional variable, C (Figure 3.1, right).

We now have a rich enough diagram (Figure 3.1, right) to introduce some terminology: Z in this causal DAG is generally considered a *confounder* of the $X{\rightarrow}Y$

Box 3.3

What Variables Do We Include in a DAG?

How do we decide what variables to include in a causal DAG? Chiefly, we rely on prior causal knowledge—our substantive background knowledge—to decide on these variables (Greenland et al., 1999; Robins, 2000).

Many investigators, however, believe incorrectly that we should do this by consulting our data Consider again the system shown in Figure 3.1 (center), where we wish to estimate the causal effect of X on Y and so the base of our diagram is $X{\rightarrow}Y$. If we are to consult our data, then we might check the data to see if there is an association observed between Z and X: if there is, then we should include Z and draw an arrow between Z and X on our DAG. The critical problem with this approach is that arrows in the DAG are *explicitly causal*: so, in order to know whether there ought to be an arrow from Z to X in the DAG, we first have to assess whether there is a causal effect of Z on X. To do so, we would now need to consider a new causal diagram, the base of which is $Z{\rightarrow}X$. Perhaps we believe that Q belongs on the $Z{\rightarrow}X$ diagram? Well, first we need to assess the causal effect $Q{\rightarrow}Z$. And so on.

The "turtles all the way down" nature of this process is partly why this is not the way we select additional variables to include in a causal DAG, but instead rely on prior causal knowledge to decide how to construct the DAG (Robins, 2000).

relationship and compromises exchangeability if we wish to estimate the effect of X on Y. Specifically, Z is a confounder because it sits on an open backdoor path (see Section 3.5.1).

C is called a *collider* on the path $X{\rightarrow}C{\leftarrow}Y$ because two arrowheads collide ($\rightarrow\leftarrow$) in node C; we will explain colliders later, but they should be sharply distinguished from confounders.

Finally, M is called a *mediator* on the path $X{\rightarrow}M{\rightarrow}Y$. M mediates the $X{\rightarrow}Y$ relationship, in that part of the effect of X on Y flows through M (follow the arrows!). Understanding that M is a mediator of the $X{\rightarrow}Y$ relationship allows us to distinguish several types of causal effects. The *total effect* of X on Y comprises two pathways: the pathway $X{\rightarrow}Y$ and the pathway $X{\rightarrow}M{\rightarrow}Y$. The *direct effect of X on Y not mediated by M* is the first of these alone; an *indirect effect of X on Y through M* is the second alone (although we do not often frame effects this way). Identification of a direct effect therefore requires us to propose one or more factors that the effect of exposure is mediated by, in this case M. There are entire textbooks (VanderWeele, 2015) dealing with mediation of causal effects; we only touch on basics here.

It is important to emphasize several points. First, the absence of an arrow between two nodes on a DAG corresponds to a strong assumption that there exists no causal relationship between those two nodes *for any individual*. This condition is called the *sharp causal null* and is a stronger assumption than the average causal null. An average null effect could result from a cancelling of positive and negative individual effects. In Figure 3.1 (right), for example, the absence of an arrow from Z to M is a strong assumption that Z does not affect M for any individual. Since it is frequently difficult to recognize things (in this case, arrows) that are absent, this represents a substantial cognitive tripping hazard with the use of DAGs.

Second, DAGs are scale-independent: the same DAG applies whether you are considering a risk difference or a risk ratio, for example. And, as such, DAGs are of somewhat limited utility when considering effect measure modification (see Chapter 5 and Chapter 6).

Finally, we noted earlier that no causal loops are allowed: this is to preserve temporality in assessment of causal effects from a DAG. For example, it is plausible that weight affects a decision to start smoking and that initiation of smoking may then affect future weight. But if this causal chain is expressed as a diagram like Figure 3.2 (upper panel), in which same variable (Weight) appears twice, then the causal diagram appears to violate temporality. Weight is measured at a point in time, and it is not possible for future smoking to affect weight in the past.

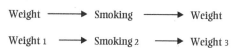

Figure 3.2 A pseudo-directed acyclic graph (DAG) without time-indexing, in which weight appears twice (*upper*); a DAG with time-indexing (*lower*), which resolves the issue.

DAGs can address this problem by time-indexing nodes: thus, the lower panel of Figure 3.2 expresses the underlying ideas with greater clarity (and without an implied causal loop).

Next we describe types of systematic error, frequently using DAGs to illustrate these concepts. This might be a good moment for you to refresh your understanding of the differences between systematic and random error (Chapter 1).

3.5 THE VARIETIES OF SYSTEMATIC ERROR

In this book, we divide the types of systematic error into four types: confounding bias, missing data bias, selection bias, and measurement error (or information bias; misclassification is a special case of this). There are certainly ways to quibble with this taxonomy.[5] Nonetheless, we view these categories as useful for introducing these concepts. We use causal DAGs to illustrate several of these biases and to expand and illustrate additional concepts. Informally, by "bias" we mean any difference between the true causal effect and the expected value of the causal effect estimated in our data, where by "expected" we mean "not due to chance alone."

As with the causal identification conditions, it is unlikely that all these ideas will be fully transparent to you the first time you encounter this material, in part because these concepts are difficult and may require multiple exposures. Another factor is that several of these biases—especially confounding—are concepts which are clarified by comparing their occurrence between study designs. Confounding in particular will generally not occur in a randomized trial (though this depends in part on what analysis is performed using trial data; see Chapter 5) but *will* generally arise in an observational cohort study (see Chapter 6). Likewise, selection bias may be more understandable after comparing and contrasting observational cohort studies (again, Chapter 6) with case-control studies (Chapter 7).

Thus, we believe that the best way to learn these concepts is to *iterate*: read the following section; read on in the book; and then, when you encounter these ideas again, circle back to this section (and this chapter as a whole) and refresh yourself on these ideas. Thus, in the remainder of this section, we seek (i) to introduce these ideas so you will have a basis for understanding these ideas when they arise later in the work (especially in Chapters 5–7) and (ii) provide a reference for you to come back to when reading those chapters to clarify these concepts.

3.5.1 Confounding Bias

Confounding bias is what is nearly always meant by the statement "correlation is not causation" and is one name for a lack of *exchangeability*, specifically nonexchangeability due to the imbalance of (typically) causes of the outcome

---

5. Increasingly, there is interest in casting all these systematic errors as problems of missing data, in part through the lens of missing data being the "fundamental problem of causal inference." See Westreich et al. (2015) for further discussion.

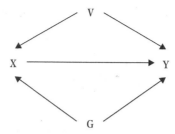

Figure 3.3 A directed acyclic graph for the effect of X on Y with two confounders (V and G).

across levels of the exposure. To be free of confounding bias, the only association between the exposure and the outcome must be due to the exposure itself, whose effect we wish to estimate. Confounding variables create such other associations between the exposure and the outcome: for example, in Figure 3.3, V creates an association between X and Y which is not the causal effect of X on Y. Such a situation maps neatly to our informal understanding of exchangeability: if V causes people to be exposed ($V{\to}X$) and V causes the outcome ($V{\to}Y$), then the pre-exposure risk of Y among those with $X = 1$ is likely to be different from the pre-exposure risk of Y among those with $X = 0$.

The classic (but problematic) definition of confounding states that a confounder is a variable which is (approximately) associated with the exposure and outcome and not caused by the exposure. This definition leaves room for subtle errors, especially those involving colliders (e.g., M-diagrams; Greenland, 2003). Addressing confounding—identifying confounders—from the perspective of causal DAGs solves several problems with more classic definitions of confounding although not without introducing additional complications.

Using a DAG, we identify the confounding variables—the variables that are leading to nonexchangeability—in the following steps (Greenland, Robins, & Pearl, 1999):

1. Remove all arrows that begin at the exposure.
2. Identify the backdoor paths: that is, paths which
   a. begin with an arrow *into the exposure*, and
   b. end with an arrow *into the outcome*.
3. For each backdoor path, determine whether the path is open or closed. Paths are open unless
   a. they contain one or more colliders, and
   b. we have not conditioned on those colliders (see below, and section 3.5.3).
4. All open backdoor paths are considered confounding paths; all variables on such paths (except the exposure and outcome) are considered confounders.

We have now identified all open backdoor paths, and thus confounders, in our diagram. We then achieve independence of the exposure and the outcome by "controlling" or "adjusting" for confounding variables, thus "closing" those otherwise open paths. What does it mean to control confounding, in practice? We might mean, for example, "include the confounder in a regression model" or "account for the confounder using standardization": we return to these ideas later in this book (Chapter 6). Here, we focus on the decision of which variables we will adjust for. We add that if we condition on a collider (3b, in the steps above) we open an otherwise closed path, a concept we explain further below (see Selection Bias).

Consider a few examples. In Figure 3.3, we would begin by removing the arrow from X to Y. This leaves two backdoor paths, both open ($X \leftarrow V \rightarrow Y$ and $X \leftarrow G \rightarrow Y$): to close all backdoor paths, we would need to control (again, for now we do not specify how we will do this) for V and G.

In Figure 3.4, removing the X to Y arrow leaves two paths. There is one backdoor path ($\underline{X} \leftarrow Z \rightarrow Y$) and one closed path containing a collider ($X \leftarrow T \rightarrow S \leftarrow Y$; remember that S is a collider on this path because the arrowheads from T and Y "collide" in that node). To close all backdoor paths in Figure 3.4, we would have to condition on Z, but we can leave the $X \leftarrow T \rightarrow S \leftarrow Y$ path alone, as it closed by the collider. If we were to condition on S, we would *open* this path.

Finally, in Figure 3.5, there is a single open path ($X \leftarrow Q \rightarrow E \rightarrow Y$): to close this path, we can condition on Q, or on E, or on both Q and E. In this last example, there are three *sufficient* sets of covariates [Q; E; Q and E]; controlling for *any of these three sets* will remove the confounding of the $X \rightarrow Y$ relationship.

Of critical importance is that we can never know whether a causal DAG has fully captured the real causal process, including all confounders of the causal relationship we want to estimate. It is always possible that, for a given DAG, there might be a variable (often designated U for unknown or unmeasured) which (for example) has arrows into both X and Y and therefore confounds their relationship. If such a U exists, then controlling for confounding based on the DAG will not deal with all biases of the causal relationship under study. It is in general impossible to rule out the existence of such a variable—except in an intention-to-treat analysis of a properly conducted randomized trial (see Chapter 5). Finally, as a note, we remind you that this is just a very preliminary introduction to DAGs. We will discuss these methods further later in this book, but the book as a whole

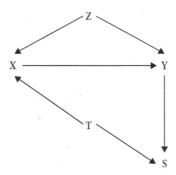

Figure 3.4 A more complicated confounding structure.

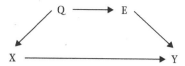

Figure 3.5 A trapezoidal directed acyclic graph showing a single confounding path with two variables on it.

is only an introduction to these methods. More details can be found in works by Hernán and Robins (Hernán & Robins, 2019) and Pearl (1995, 2009).

3.5.2 Missing Data

Missing data bias results from lack of complete information on exposure, outcomes, or covariates in a study. For example, if, in a study of 100 participants, 20 did not have an exposure status recorded, we would describe that situation as *missing exposure data*.

Generally, we think of missing data in three main categories: missing completely at random, missing at random, and missing not at random. *Missing completely at random* (MCAR) data are missing exactly as you think: completely at random, as if the data which are *not* missing are a simple random sample of the full data. If 10% of outcome data are missing completely at random, for example, it is the same as saying that for each individual we rolled a fair 10-sided die, and, if we roll a 7, then we replace their outcome with a "missing" indicator. Data might be missing completely at random if a gust of wind caused a stack of unordered test results on paper to be blown away, and some sheets of paper were swept into a lake and destroyed before they could be recovered.

Data which are truly MCAR are rare: more common are data *missing at random* (MAR). MAR is a confusing name, sounding too much like MCAR to be clearly distinguished by the language. MAR indicates data which are missing independent of the missing data itself, conditional on the observed data for each individual. For example, if exposure is fully observed in all participants, and outcome is missing in 10% of participants who are exposed and 20% of participants who are unexposed, and missingness does not depend on any other variables, then we would conclude that outcome data are MAR.

Data *missing not at random* (MNAR) are missing data which are neither MCAR nor MAR, and therefore those where the missingness depends on the unobserved value of the missing variable itself. Age would be MNAR if age were missing more often in older people than in younger people.

3.5.2.1 ANALYSIS WITH MISSING DATA

The most common way of addressing missing data is to perform what is called a *complete case analysis*, in which only those observations which have full data available are analyzed. For example, consider an analysis of the effect of exposure X on outcome Y controlling for covariates Z_1, Z_2, and Z_3. Complete case analysis

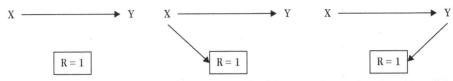

Figure 3.6 Three causal diagrams showing causal mechanisms for missing data. The box around $R = 1$ indicates that we have restricted analysis to participants who are not missing (who Responded). In the left panel, probability of response is independent of both exposure X and outcome Y; in the center panel, probability of response is caused by exposure; in the right panel, probability of response is caused by the outcome.

would include only those individuals who had no missing data for *any* of those five variables.

Such an approach, however, may lead to biased estimates. Under what circumstances does a complete case analysis result in bias? Broadly, this is a product not of *information* structure (e.g., MAR/MNAR distinctions) but of *causal* structure. In particular, we can have situations of both MAR and MNAR in which there is *no* bias in complete case analysis and also situations of both MAR and MNAR in which there *is* bias in complete case analysis. However, since MCAR data are independent of the outcome (and all other observed variables), complete case analysis of MCAR data is generally unbiased. (Daniel, Kenward, Cousens, & De Stavola, 2012).

We demonstrate some of these issues in simple examples, using the three DAGs in Figure 3.6 and accompanying data in Table 3.2. In Figure 3.6, $R = 1$ with a box around it indicates that we have restricted analysis to individuals

Table 3.2 FULL (TOP) AND PARTIALLY OBSERVED (BOTTOM) DATA RELATED TO FIGURE 3.6 (LEFT, CENTER, RIGHT PANELS) TO ILLUSTRATE THAT DATA MISSING NOT AT RANDOM NEED NOT LEAD TO BIAS IN SIMPLE ANALYSIS

Full	$Y = 1$	$Y = 0$	Total	Risk
$X = 1$	200	800	1,000	0.2
$X = 0$	100	900	1,000	0.1
Left	$Y = 1$	$Y = 0$	Total	Risk
$X = 1$	160	640	800	0.2
$X = 0$	80	720	800	0.1
Center	$Y = 1$	$Y = 0$	Total	Risk
$X = 1$	100	400	500	0.2
$X = 0$	80	720	800	0.1
Right	$Y = 1$	$Y = 0$	Total	Risk
$X = 1$	180	400	580	0.31
$X = 0$	90	450	540	0.17

who have no missingness on X or Y (R for response). In the left panel, R is independent of both X and Y. In Table 3.2, the top 2×2 table (labeled Full) is example data without any missingness, and the second 2×2 table (labeled Left) corresponds to Figure 3.6 (left). In Table 3.2 (Left), 20% of the full table is missing in every cell, equally: so instead of 200 exposed disease cases, we see 160, and we estimate the same exposure-specific risks (and same risk difference) as in the Full data.

In the center panel of Figure 3.6, things are more complicated: there is an open path from R to Y ($R \leftarrow X \rightarrow Y$). The 2×2 table in Table 3.2 (Center) shows missingness which differs by level of X; 50% of those with $X = 1$ are missing, but only 20% of those with $X = 0$. In this table, we see that the exposure-specific risks are estimated accurately from the data, and therefore we can estimate the correct risk difference from those exposure-specific risks. This is because the open path between R and Y is closed conditional on X (see below).

In the right panel of Figure 3.6, we show missingness differential by level of Y, because $Y \rightarrow R$. The last 2×2 table in Table 3.2 (Right) shows missingness which differs by level of Y: 10% of those with $Y = 1$ are missing, and 50% of those with $Y = 0$. The exposure-specific risks here are incorrect and so is the risk difference (about 0.14), showing the bias that can arise when missingness is caused by the outcome as in the right panel of Figure 3.6.

We make three brief points. First, note that there is no bias in the risk difference for Figure 3.6 (center) but there is bias in the risk difference for Figure 3.6 (right), as is evident in Table 3.2. Now recognize that $X \rightarrow R$ in Figure 3.6 could mean that the true value of X is the cause of missingness in X (which would mean the data are MNAR) or of missingness in Y (which would mean the data are MAR). Similarly, recognize that $Y \rightarrow R$ in Figure 3.6 could mean that the true value of Y is the cause of missingness in Y (which would mean the data are MNAR) or of missingness in X (which would mean the data are MAR). Thus, we have demonstrated that whether data are MAR or MNAR does not tell you whether or not there is bias in complete case analysis. (Daniel, Kenward, Cousens, & De Stavola, 2012).

Second, key to understanding causal diagrams for missing data is the independence of missingness and the outcome (Daniel, Kenward, Cousens, & De Stavola, 2012). For example, the reason there is no bias from Figure 3.6 (center) is that when we condition on X (i.e., within levels of X), there is no association between missingness and the outcome. On the other hand, analysis of the total incidence of the outcome (which is *not* conditional on X) in this diagram will be biased: the total incidence of $Y = 1$ in the Center table $((100 + 80)/(500 + 800))$ *is* biased compared to the full table $((200 + 100)/(1,000 + 1,000))$. And third, and closely related, all these issues become much more complex when confounders are added to diagrams: such complexities are beyond the scope of this book and are the subject of ongoing methodological work. Here, we want you to come away with the basic understanding that MAR and MNAR are not the same as biased or unbiased in complete case analysis, as we have demonstrated.

So what, then, is the use of MAR and MNAR distinctions? They tell us when— under missing data—we can correct for any bias that exists or improve the

Missingness category	Complete case analysis biased?	If complete case is biased, can existing analytic methods fully fix it?
MCAR	No	NA (but these methods can improve precision)
MAR	Maybe, depends on causal structure	Yes in general
MNAR	Maybe, depends on causal structure	No in general (*may* reduce bias, but not eliminate)

Note that we assume no measurement error throughout.

precision of our estimates using more advanced analytic techniques such as *multiple imputation* (Little & Rubin, 2002) or *inverse probability weighting* (Hernán & Robins, 2019). Specifically, multiple imputation and other methods generally depend on data being MAR (or MCAR) rather than MNAR. When data are MNAR, such techniques cannot be expected to eliminate all bias due to missing data. Of course, just as we can never know whether uncontrolled confounding is present (e.g., if we have left a critical covariate out of our DAG), we can never know for certain whether missing data are missing at random or not at random (i.e., are missing at least in part due to the unobserved true values of the given variables). We summarize some of this information in Table 3.3.

Therefore, in the left and center panels of Figure 3.6, complete case analysis for the effect of X on Y (again, analysis of only those participants with no missing data on any variable) will be unbiased due to the missing data; however, multiple imputation, if possible, might improve the statistical efficiency (i.e., the precision) of the estimate. In the right panel of Figure 3.6, the complete case analysis will be biased, but multiple imputation (or a related technique) might be able to reduce the bias if the true value of Y is leading only X to be missing. We omit discussion of how to implement multiple imputation and inverse probability of missingness weighting; readers can find such discussions elsewhere.

3.5.3 Selection Bias

In epidemiology, the term "selection bias" means several things depending on context. These include bias resulting from the noninclusion of study subjects in analysis, for example, because of loss-to-follow-up (out-selection); bias resulting from conditioning or restricting on a collider (collider selection bias; Hernán, Hernández-Díaz, & Robins, 2004); and bias resulting from the selection of subjects into a study (in-selection bias, sampling bias, or generalizability bias). In this work we distinguish the three while acknowledging that all three are reasonably called "selection bias" by epidemiologists (Hernán, 2017).

The first form of selection bias we discuss is *analytic selection bias*, which includes selection bias due to loss to follow-up and which overlaps with issues of missing data in some cases. In particular, when we analyze only cases with no missing data (described earlier as complete case analysis) the two can coincide: cases with no missing data are *selected* for analysis; those with missing data (leading to non-analysis) are not selected. As with missing data, we can analyze whether selection is likely to lead to bias by using DAGs (such as Figure 3.6) and sometimes adjust for selection using analytic techniques (see Table 3.3).

The second type of selection bias is due to conditioning or restricting on a collider, called *collider bias*. Recall that a collider is a variable which is jointly caused by two additional variables (e.g., node C in Figure 3.7). For example, your steps may be wet because it rained or because the sprinkler system has a timer—the wetness (or not) of the steps is a collider for rain and the sprinkler. While X affects C and Y also affects C ($X \rightarrow C \leftarrow Y$) it is possible that there is no direct relationship (or arrow) between X and Y, as in Figure 3.7 (left).

Another example: if smoking affects risk of heart attack and so do the genetics of cholesterol metabolism, there may not be a direct relationship between genetics and smoking. But *among those who have a heart attack* (where $C = 1$, a form of conditioning on the node C) there may be a relationship between the two nodes. This is because among those who have a heart attack, there is often a reason; among those *who have a heart attack* ($C = 1$) *who do not smoke* ($X = 0$), those reasons are more likely to be genetic than for in others in the population. Thus, in those individuals who have had a heart attack, knowing that they do not smoke raises the probability that they have some genetic susceptibility to heart attack. This induced relationship between smoking and genetics after conditioning on heart attack is sometimes informally shown on a DAG as a dotted line between X and Y. This is illustrated in Figure 3.7, in which, unconditional on C, there is no relationship between X and Y (left); once we condition on C (right; the box around C indicates we are holding C constant at any level), we induce a noncausal association (shown as the dotted line) between X and Y.

Collider bias is sometimes considered a form of selection bias (Hernán et al., 2004); but see also (Hernán, 2017) though others find this use of "selection" somewhat confusing. Frequently, to "select" something is to pick that something out

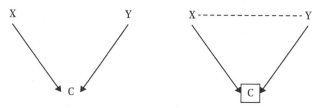

Figure 3.7 Two causal diagrams illustrating the effects of conditioning on a collider. On the left, X and Y have a common effect, C; on the right, conditioning on C leads to a spurious connection between X and Y (that could be misinterpreted as a causal effect of X on Y).

while leaving other things behind. While some forms of collider bias (particularly, *restricting* on a collider) coincide with this connotative usage, other uses (conditioning on C in $X \rightarrow C \leftarrow Y$ as in the right panel of Figure 3.7) do not match up with typical and widespread uses of the word "selection," leading to some confusion. Whatever it is called, however, conditioning on a collider can lead to dramatically incorrect study conclusions, including several issues that are otherwise considered "paradoxes" (Hernández-Díaz, Schisterman, & Hernán, 2006; Stovitz, Banack, & Kaufman, 2018).

The last common use of selection bias is *in-selection bias*, which is a problem of the generalizability of findings from a study to some external target population (see Chapter 9 for further discussion of target populations). This might occur if, for example, the results of your study vary by age, and the distribution of age differs between your study sample and your target population. While calling this a kind of selection bias is a perfectly reasonable approach and matches up well with broad usage of "selection," in this work we will distinguish this manifestation of selection bias by referring to it as *generalizability-bias* or *sampling bias*.

3.5.4 Information Bias

Here, we consider "information bias" and "measurement error" to be interchangeable terms and "misclassification" to be closely related. Errors of this type can arise for numerous reasons—and can lead to bias even when the error is entirely random.

Information bias is in some ways easiest to understand when considering a two-category variable—for example, "exposed" and "not exposed"—and how individuals in one group may be mislabeled as belonging to the other group. This is a special case of measurement error we call *misclassification*. Consider the 2×2 table shown in Table 3.4 (top), which we presume tells us the truth about the world: in particular, that the risk difference (for some fixed time period) comparing exposed to unexposed is $0.10 - 0.05 = 0.05$. Now suppose that we have a flawed test for assessing exposure, which randomly misclassifies 20% of all truly exposed individuals as unexposed (i.e., the test has a sensitivity of 80%, see Chapter 4). However, this test never misclassifies the unexposed people. In this case, we would observe a table in which 20% of the truly exposed individuals (with their outcome risk of 10%) are analyzed *as if they*

Table 3.4 AN ILLUSTRATION OF INFORMATION BIAS

	Outcome	No outcome	Total	Risk
Exposed	100	900	1,000	0.1000
Unexposed	50	950	1,000	0.0500
	Outcome	No outcome	Total	Risk
Exposed	80	720	800	0.1000
Unexposed	70	1,130	1,200	0.0583

are unexposed: this is the equivalent of moving 200 individuals total, of whom 20 experienced the outcome, from the exposed to the unexposed group and reanalyzing the data (Table 3.4, bottom). This leads to the overall risk of the outcome in the unexposed group being estimated at about 5.8%, rather than 5%—and that in turn leads to a biased estimate of the causal effect, which will now be estimated as $0.100 - 0.058 = {\sim}4.2\%$ instead of 5%. Thus, misclassification of the exposure leads to bias in this case; we encourage you to create your own example misclassifying the outcome (e.g., taking 10% of those within the Outcome column and shifting them to the No outcome column, the same way in each row) to see what happens.

Table 3.4 presents an example of *nondifferential misclassification of the exposure*, which in the case of two categories will tend (on average) to move the effect estimate toward the null value of the effect in question (i.e., toward 0 for a risk difference, or 1 for a risk ratio). The misclassification here is "nondifferential" because the *probability of being misclassified is independent of the true outcome status*. The bias toward the null (e.g., a risk difference closer to zero) is due to the fact that moving individuals randomly from exposed to unexposed (or vice versa, or both at once) will tend (on average) to make the two groups more similar. At one possible extreme, when the exposed/unexposed label is assigned at random, irrespective of true exposure, the two groups will have the same proportion of exposed and unexposed participants, and we will detect no differences between them. It should not surprise us, therefore, that as two groups become more similar due to misclassification, the differences between them tend to grow smaller.

This idea that "nondifferential misclassification of the exposure will lead to bias toward the null" is widely repeated and often misunderstood in its particulars, and so it is worth examining more closely. First, and most critically, this is a statement about averages: while the direction of the bias is predictable, in any given example or dataset the realization of nondifferential misclassification is subject to random as well as systematic error. Such random error may lead to data in which supposedly nondifferential misclassification leads to bias away from the null (Jurek, Greenland, Maldonado, & Church, 2005). As well, if there are more than two exposure categories, the direction of bias resulting from nondifferential exposure misclassification is unpredictable. Finally, when misclassification is *differential*, all bets are off: if (for example) exposure was misclassified only among those who experienced the outcome, or at different rates among those who had the outcome and those who did not, the direction of bias would be generally unpredictable.

Information bias generally can result from a number of processes, including systematic bias in collection of information or faulty instrumentation. It is an important form of systematic error, especially because measurement error that occurs completely at random can introduce bias into effect estimates. For example, if random noise makes two distinct groups look more similar, then comparisons between those groups may be attenuated. We describe approaches to addressing information bias in Chapter 4.

3.5.5 Internal and External Validity

Having now discussed both the notion of a study sample compared to a target population and the biases which can arise, we can discuss the notions of both *internal validity* and *external validity*. Recall from Chapter 1 that *validity* is defined as a lack of bias, or lack of systematic error such as those just described. Assuming for the moment that we have no random error, we can define internal validity as the condition in which we have no bias in our estimate of causal effect within the study sample: that is, when the *estimated causal effect in the study sample* is equal to the *true causal effect in the study sample*. This condition is shown more formally at the end of the Appendix to this chapter.

In contrast, there is external validity when the *true effect in the study sample* is equal to the *true effect in the target population*, or alternatively when "the [true] causal relationship holds over variation in persons" (Shadish, Cook, & Campbell, 2002, p. 472) and perhaps other factors. In cases where the target population is exactly equal to the study sample, there is perfect external validity. For the most part in this book, we focus on estimating *internally valid* causal effects, but we discuss external validity in several places as well. Discussion of the relationship between internal and external validity is ongoing in the methodological literature (see Westreich, et al., 2019).

3.6 MEASURES OF CAUSAL EFFECT

3.6.1 Measures of Effect

We now briefly return to the measures of association we described in Chapter 2. Recall that all the measures of association discussed in Chapter 2 can be estimated without attention to the causal identification conditions and biases/systematic errors noted earlier, but then the resulting estimates can only be interpreted as associations and not as estimate of causal effect.

For example, we can estimate a risk difference from an observed 2 × 2 table of data even if exchangeability is not met in the data, specifically if the exposure–outcome relationship is confounded. However, if the exposure–outcome relationship is confounded, we can only interpret that risk difference as an *association* but not as a *causal effect*. If we wish to interpret an estimated risk difference as an estimate of a causal effect, we should be prepared to defend why we think the risk difference in question meets the causal identification conditions noted earlier or can be considered causal for some other reasons (e.g., meets an alternative set of identification conditions). Earlier, we showed how application of some of these conditions allows us to connect the association with the estimated causal effect for the risk difference; similar processes can be applied to the risk ratio, odds ratio, and other measures of association explored in Chapter 2.

Now we discuss two measures which were *not* covered in Chapter 2 because both can be viewed as more *inherently* causal measures and cannot be easily or sensibly interpreted in terms of association alone. These are the *number needed to treat* (NNT) and the *population attributable fraction*: these should be calculated,

Table 3.5 A 2 × 2 TABLE FOR THE EFFECT OF TREATMENT
VERSUS NO TREATMENT ON 5-YEAR RISK OF MYOCARDIAL
INFARCTION, WITH CALCULATED RISKS

	MI	No MI	Total	Risk
Treatment	60	940	1,000	0.06
No treatment	100	900	1,000	0.10
Total	160	1840	2,000	0.08

reported, and interpreted only when we can make a reasoned argument that they can be interpreted causally—and otherwise only with extreme caution.[6] (See Chapter 9 for further discussion of both measures.)

3.6.2 Number Needed to Treat

Consider a new pharmacotherapy ("Treatment") to prevent heart attack (myocardial infarction, MI) in older adults, in a study lasting 5 years. Data for this study are shown in Table 3.5, where those not taking the treatment have a 10% risk of MI over 5 years, while those taking the treatment over that period have a 6% risk. We could use these numbers to calculate the 5-year risk difference associated with treatment (0.06 − 0.10 = −0.04) and likewise we could calculate a risk or odds ratio.

Suppose instead we wish to ask "How many untreated people would we have to treat in order to prevent one MI?" This is the *number needed to treat*, and it is self-evidently about causality: we are asking not about associations, but about the likely effects of making a change in the world by treating people with a specific drug.

The NNT is calculated as simply the reciprocal of the absolute value of the risk difference. Since the risk difference is −0.04, its absolute value is 0.04, and $0.04^{-1} = 25$: thus, we would have to treat 25 untreated people to prevent one MI over 5 years (note the inclusion of the time period in the interpretation, much like the risk difference itself requires). Convention is often that we round the NNT up to the nearest integer because we cannot intervene on a portion of a person. However, this approach is also considered conservative.

In this case, the treatment was protective; when a treatment or exposure is harmful, we can calculate a number in the same way but often describe that value as a *number needed to harm* (NNH). However, NNT versus NNH distinctions are ultimately a matter of both subject matter convention and clarity in explanation.

One key caveat to the NNT is that it can be calculated whenever a risk difference is available—calculated, but not always interpreted. If there is no obvious "treatment" for the exposure under study—or the treatment is vague or ambiguously defined—then presentation of the NNT may be contraindicated (though

6. Although the published literature is replete with uses of both measures in which neither explicit causal arguments nor such caution is brought to bear.

we might still want to calculate a "number needed to expose" or other analogous measure, depending on the circumstances. We discuss this further in Chapter 9.

3.6.3 Population Attributable Effects

Let's return to an example from Chapter 2, that of the environmental contaminant (e.g., a chemical spill): suppose we were interested not in the difference in risk, but in prevention. Suppose we are considering what impact it would have if we had been able to prevent the contaminant from affecting anyone, such that all those who were exposed were instead not exposed. As with the NNT, this idea is inherently causal: it imagines a world in which we can intervene to remove the harmful exposure and estimate the effect of doing so from the data in front of us (as in this chapter).

Recall that in our initial example (Table 2.2) we stated that we enrolled 2,000 participants into our study; 1,000 of whom were exposed and 1,000 of whom were unexposed. The 5-year risk difference can still be calculated here as 0.04 or 4%. But the risk difference does not answer our question, which was "what impact would it have if we could move all those in the exposed category to have the risk profile of the unexposed category?" Unlike the risk difference, this is about comparing the overall risk in this population (calculated in the "Total" row as 0.050) to the overall risk in this population if the 1,000 exposed individuals had not been exposed.

Had, counter-to-fact, the 1,000 exposed individuals not been exposed, what would their risk be? If we assume exchangeability between the exposed and unexposed individuals here (which might be reasonable if the exposure was essentially distributed at random in the affected population), then the exposed individuals, had they not been exposed, could be assumed to have experienced the same risk as those who were not exposed in fact: that risk being 0.030. Thus, if all the originally exposed and originally unexposed people experienced a risk of 0.030 (Table 3.6), then the total population risk would be 0.030. We could then contrast the original total population risk (0.050) to the total population risk if all exposed participants had instead been unexposed (0.030).

Table 3.6 A PAIR OF 2 × 2 TABLES: THE FIRST RECAPITULATES TABLE 2.2; THE SECOND SHOWS RISK IF ALL EXPOSED INDIVIDUALS WERE MOVED TO UNEXPOSED

	Cancer	No cancer	Total	Risk
Exposed	70	930	1,000	0.070
Unexposed	30	970	1,000	0.030
Total	100	1,900	2,000	0.05
Still exposed	0	0	0	0.070
Was exposed, now unexposed	30	970	1,000	0.030
Unexposed	30	970	1,000	0.030
Total	60	1,940	2,000	0.030

Broadly, such a comparison is called a *population attributable effect*; the most common of such effects is the *population attributable fraction* (PAF). The PAF is generally defined as the percentage of outcomes which can be attributed to the exposure—and thus, the percentage of outcomes which would disappear if, counter to fact, the exposure had not occurred or was removed entirely. In this case, it is calculated as the difference between the risk in the original total population and the risk in the population in which everyone is unexposed (0.050 − 0.030), divided by the total risk in the original population (0.050): this comes out to 0.40. That is, 40% of the total outcome risk could be removed if we could have prevented exposure in all those exposed. Alternatively, we can calculate the PAF from the risk ratio (RR) and exposure prevalence ($Pr(E = 1)$):

$$\frac{Pr(E=1)\times(RR-1)}{Pr(E=1)\times(RR-1)+1}$$

In this case, $Pr(E = 1)$ is 0.5, and $RR = 2.33$, and so this equation becomes (0.5 × (2.33 − 1)) / (0.5 × (2.33 − 1) + 1) = 0.6667/1.6667 = 0.40, the same answer as we estimated immediately above. As this equation implies, we should expect the PAF to change with the prevalence of exposure. You might wish to create a numerical example exploring this phenomenon using a spreadsheet.

We can also calculate a *population attributable risk difference*, which is simply the numerator above: 0.050 − 0.030 = 0.020. This is the absolute difference in risk we would see over five years in the whole population if we had prevented exposure in all those exposed. These uses of "population attributable" correspond to what Greenland and Robins previously called "excess" cases of disease (Greenland & Robins, 1988; Rockhill, Newman, & Weinberg, 1998). As these authors note, we have omitted consideration of those for whom the absence of the exposure would have moved the incidence of the outcomes later in time and yet still within the follow-up period (within 5 years, in our preceding example).

As with the NNT, a population attributable effect (and our descriptions of it) is inherently causal: one cannot, in a reasonable use of language, "attribute" an outcome to something which did not cause that outcome. In light of some differences in terminology, what seems most critical for a user of these methods is to be clear that they are being used to estimate a causal effect. Then the user can be precise as to what causal effect they believe their calculation to be estimating, with attention to the causal identification conditions as well as possible additional considerations (see Chapter 9).

One final caution on PAFs is that—because many outcomes are caused by more than one factor (see Section 3.7.2)—PAFs can sum to more than 1 for the same outcome. As a trivial example, no one can die of AIDS without having HIV infection; thus, by definition, the PAF for the exposure of HIV and the outcome of death from AIDS is 100%. But because people die with AIDS for all sorts of additional reasons as well—having HIV is necessary but not sufficient to die of AIDS—the PAFs for HIV infection and (for example) tuberculosis infection will sum to more than 1.

3.7 OTHER MODELS OF CAUSALITY AND CAUSAL INFERENCE

In this text, we focus on potential outcomes and causal DAGs as approaches to causal effect estimation. However, historically, numerous other approaches have been taken to causal inference and causal effect estimation. Here, we briefly describe a few of these.

3.7.1 The Hill Lecture

Perhaps the most famous of these are the "causal criteria" of Sir Austin Bradford Hill. A lecture given by Hill, the summary of which was published in *Proceedings of the Royal Society of Medicine* in 1965, described nine criteria that might help us distinguish whether a particular factor is a cause of disease (Hill, 1965). He listed the following guideposts: strength of association, consistency of association (which he meant in a broad sense, not the narrow causal identification condition noted earlier), specificity of association, temporality, biological gradient (such as a dose–response relationship), plausibility, coherence (with known facts), experiment, and analogy.

Notably, these guideposts have been repeatedly used as a checklist to determine whether an association is causal, despite Hill's specific caution that he did not believe:

> We can usefully lay down some hard-and-fast rules of evidence that must be obeyed before we accept cause and effect. None of my nine viewpoints can bring indisputable evidence for or against the cause-and-effect hypothesis and none can be required as a *sine qua non.*

(Many would argue that temporality is indeed a *sine qua non*!)

Again, we are restricting ourselves in this book to causal effect estimation, which is not the same as causal inference (Greenland, 2017): in particular, the latter is a much wider field, and we do not rule out Hill's guidelines as potentially useful for larger scale considerations of causal inference. Ultimately, Hill's goal was in deciding when sufficient evidence has accumulated to drive action to guard health: a decision which involves more than causal effect estimation. In this work, we rely on a combination of the potential outcome framework and causal diagrams to help guide causal effect estimation.

3.7.2 Sufficient Component Causal Framework ("Causal Pies")

This model of causality was introduced by Rothman in 1976 (1976, 2012) and is very helpful in thinking about "multicausality": the idea that events occur only in the presence of multiple causal factors. Specifically, a particular case of disease generally has many contributing causes, all of which are necessary to that particular case. For example, person Z was eating dinner when they suddenly suffered a heart attack; the restaurant called paramedics but person Z died before

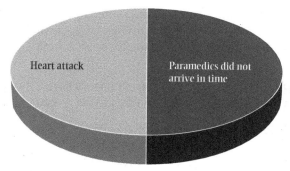

Figure 3.8 A causal pie representing one set of causes for a death.

they could arrive. Here, perhaps the necessary causes of the outcome of death include the heart attack and also the fact that the paramedics did not arrive in time (Figure 3.8). Had either of those two causes been absent (i.e., had the heart attack not occurred or had the paramedics arrived in time), the outcome (death) would not have occurred. Alternatively, had there been a heart attack and yet a timely paramedic arrival—or no heart attack, but a late paramedic arrival—then person Z would not have died. (It is, of course, notable that without the heart attack, a paramedic arrival would have been very strange—but nonetheless Z would still be alive.)

In this framework, each instance of the outcome gets its own pie, reflecting the causes that were necessary to that case of the outcome: so a different death might be attributed to heart attack and lack of a phone so that the paramedics could not be called in the first place, and a third death to other factors entirely. Though we will not dwell on causal pies further, it is worth mentioning that the causal types we introduced earlier (doomed, immune, etc.) can be mapped to people who do or do not have certain component causes.

3.8 SUMMARY

There is contentious and ongoing debate about the best approach to causal effect estimation and causal inference within epidemiology. We ally ourselves with the view that both potential outcomes and causal diagrams are extremely useful in the conceptualization and estimation of quantitative causal effects: that is, in the estimation of the quantitative effect of a well-defined exposure on an outcome. This is the approach we take in this work because our goal—improving the health of populations—requires well-defined exposures and outcomes and estimates of the causal effects of interventions against those exposures. We do not make any universal claim about the applicability of this framework to causality or causal inference in general—only the estimation of quantitative causal effects.

The view of causality presented here, including potential outcomes and causal diagrams, integrated with an understanding of descriptive and predictive epidemiology (in the form of surveillance and screening, Chapter 4), key study designs (Chapters 5–8), and the causal impact framework (Chapter 9), is the best way I know to help craft (relatively!) unambiguous epidemiologic inquiries, the answers to which have high potential to improve public health.

APPENDIX: HOW CAUSAL IDENTIFICATION CONDITIONS HELP IDENTIFY CAUSAL EFFECT ESTIMATES FROM ASSOCIATIONS

Recall that we previously stated our associational risk difference as

$$\Pr(Y = 1 \mid X = 1) - \Pr(Y = 1 \mid X = 0)$$

However, we may wish to rewrite this as

$$\Pr(Y^* = 1 \mid X^* = 1) - \Pr(Y^* = 1 \mid X^* = 0)$$

to indicate that the true values of both Y and X might be measured with error. Only by assuming *no measurement error* can we return to our original statement of the associational risk difference.

We further assume *temporality* because, without assurance that X preceded Y in time, no causal interpretation of the effect of X on Y can proceed.

Now, we apply *consistency* and *exchangeability*. Recall that consistency is that *among people who were exposed*, the effect of their exposure was no different than it would have been if they had been assigned that treatment—and the same is true for the unexposed. This assumption allows us to move from the observed risk difference

$$\Pr(Y = 1 \mid X = 1) - \Pr(Y = 1 \mid X = 0)$$

one step toward the causal risk difference, as follows:

$$\Pr\left(Y^{x=1} = 1 \mid X = 1\right)$$

Now we address exchangeability: if exchangeability holds, then it is the case that *the risk of the exposed can stand in for the risk of the unexposed, if—counter to fact— the unexposed had been exposed.* If this is true, then the risk of Y under assignment to $X = 1$ estimated only among those who were observed to be treated (i.e., $\Pr(Y^{x=1} = 1)$) can stand in for the risk of Y under assignment to $X = 1$ estimated in the whole population (i.e., $\Pr(Y^{x=0} = 1 \mid X = 0) = \Pr(Y^{x=0} = 1)$). The same logic in reverse allows us to state that $\Pr(Y^{x=0} = 1 \mid X = 0) = \Pr(Y^{x=0} = 1)$. Together, these allow us to transform the expression post-consistency, namely

$$\Pr(Y^{x=1} = 1 \mid X = 1) - \Pr(Y^{x=0} = 1 \mid X = 0)$$

to the following

$$\Pr(Y^{x=1} = 1) - \Pr(Y^{x=0} = 1)$$

or simply

$$= \Pr(Y^{x=1}) - \Pr(Y^{x=0})$$

which is the average causal risk difference. Thus, when no measurement error, temporality, consistency, and exchangeability hold (or we assume them to hold, hopefully with good reason), we can interpret the observed risk difference as an estimate of the causal risk difference. In Chapter 5, we will explain how randomized trials can provide most of these conditions for us; in Chapter 6, we will explain further how to achieve conditional exchangeability.

Having presented the preceding notation, we can also use it to define internal validity. Specifically, internal validity is when the estimated causal effect in the population under study (the study sample) is exactly equal to the true causal effect in the study sample. We could express this as

$$\Pr(Y^{*} = 1 \mid X^{*} = 1) - \Pr(Y^{*} = 1 \mid X^{*} = 0) = \Pr(Y^{x=1}) - \Pr(Y^{x=0})$$

or we could be more explicit that we are in the study sample by defining $S = 1$ as the condition of being in the study sample and define internal validity as

$$\Pr(Y^{*} = 1 \mid X^{*} = 1, S = 1) - \Pr(Y^{*} = 1 \mid X^{*} = 0, S = 1)$$
$$= \Pr(Y^{x=1} \mid S = 1) - \Pr(Y^{x=0} \mid S = 1).$$

See Westreich et al. (2019) for further discussion on this and related points.

REFERENCES

Cooper, R. S. (2013). Race in biological and biomedical research. *Cold Spring Harbor Perspectives on Medicine, 3*(11). doi:10.1101/cshperspect.a008573

Daniel, R. M., Kenward, M. G., Cousens, S. N., & De Stavola, B. L. (2012). Using causal diagrams to guide analysis in missing data problems. *Statistics and Methods in Medical Research, 21*(3), 243–256. doi:10.1177/0962280210394469

Greenland, S. (2003). Quantifying biases in causal models: Classical confounding vs collider-stratification bias. *Epidemiology, 14*(3), 300–306.

Greenland, S. (2017). For and against methodologies: Some perspectives on recent causal and statistical inference debates. *European Journal of Epidemiology, 32*(1), 3–20. doi:10.1007/s10654-017-0230-6

Greenland, S., Pearl, J., & Robins, J. M. (1999). Causal diagrams for epidemiologic research. *Epidemiology, 10*(1), 37–48.

Greenland, S., & Robins, J. M. (1988). Conceptual problems in the definition and interpretation of attributable fractions. *American Journal of Epidemiology, 128*(6), 1185–1197.

Hernán, M. A. (2017). Invited commentary: Selection bias without colliders. *American Journal of Epidemiology, 185*(11), 1048–1050. doi:10.1093/aje/kwx077

Hernán, M. A., Hernández-Díaz, S., & Robins, J. M. (2004). A structural approach to selection bias. *Epidemiology, 15*(5), 615–625.

Hernán, M. A., & Robins, J. M. (2019). *Causal inference.* Boca Raton: Chapman & Hall/ CRC. Retrieved from http://www.hsph.harvard.edu/miguel-hernan/causal-inference-book/.

Hernández-Díaz, S., Schisterman, E. F., & Hernán, M. A. (2006). The birth weight "paradox" uncovered? *American Journal of Epidemiology, 164*(11), 1115–1120.

Hill, A. B. (1965). The environment and disease: Association or causation? *Proceedings of the Royal Society of Medicine, 58,* 295–300.

Holland, P. W. (1986). Statistics and causal inference. *Journal of the American Statistical Association, 81*(396), 945–960.

Jurek, A. M., Greenland, S., Maldonado, G., & Church, T. R. (2005). Proper interpretation of non-differential misclassification effects: Expectations vs observations. *International Journal of Epidemiology, 34*(3), 680–687. doi:10.1093/ije/dyi060

Kaufman, J. S., Cooper, R. S., & McGee, D. L. (1997). Socioeconomic status and health in blacks and whites: The problem of residual confounding and the resiliency of race. *Epidemiology, 8*(6), 621–628.

Keil, A. P., Mooney, S. J., Jonsson Funk, M., Cole, S. R., Edwards, J. K., & Westreich, D. (2018). Resolving an apparent paradox in doubly robust estimators. *American Journal of Epidemiology, 187*(4), 891–892. doi:10.1093/aje/kwx385

Little, R. J. A., & Rubin, D. B. (2002). *Statistical analysis with missing data* (2nd ed.). New York: John Wiley.

Maldonado, G., & Greenland, S. (2002). Estimating causal effects. *International Journal of Epidemiology, 31*(2), 422–429.

Naimi, A. I., & Balzer, L. B. (2018). Stacked generalization: An introduction to super learning. *European Journal of Epidemiology, 33*(5), 459–464. doi:10.1007/ s10654-018-0390-z

Neyman, J. (1923/1990). On the application of probability theory to agricultural experiments. Essay on principles. Section 9. *Statistical Science, 5*(4), 465–472. Trans. D. M. Dabrowska & T. P. Speed.

Pearl, J. (1995). Causal diagrams for empirical research. *Biometrika, 82*(4), 669–688.

Pearl, J. (2009). *Causality* (2nd ed.). New York: Cambridge University Press.

Porta, M. (Ed.). (2014). *A dictionary of epidemiology* (6th ed.). New York: Oxford University Press.

Robins, J. M. (2000). Data, design, and background knowledge in etiologic inference. *Epidemiology, 11*(3), 313–320.

Rockhill, B., Newman, B., & Weinberg, C. (1998). Use and misuse of population attributable fractions. *American Journal of Public Health, 88*(1), 15–19.

Rothman, K. J. (1976). Causes. *American Journal of Epidemiology, 104*(6), 587–592.

Rothman, K. J. (2012). *Epidemiology: An introduction.* New York: Oxford University Press.

Rubin, D. B. (1974). Estimating causal effects of treatments in randomized and nonrandomized studies. *Journal of Educational Psychology, 66*(5), 688–701.

Shadish, W., Cook, T., & Campbell, D. (2002). *Experimental and quasi-experimental designs for generalized causal inference.* New York: Houghton Mifflin.

Stovitz, S. D., Banack, H. R., & Kaufman, J. S. (2018). Paediatric obesity appears to lower the risk of diabetes if selection bias is ignored. *Journal of Epidemiology and Community Health*, *72*(4), 302–308. doi:10.1136/jech-2017-209985

van der Laan, M. J., & Rose, S. (2011). *Targeted learning: Causal inference for observational and experimental data.* New York: Springer.

VanderWeele, T. J. (2015). *Explanation in causal inference.* New York: Oxford University Press.

VanderWeele, T. J., & Robins, J. M. (2012). Stochastic counterfactuals and stochastic sufficient causes. *Statitistica Sinica*, *22*(1), 379–392. doi:10.5705/ss.2008.186

Westreich, D. (2017). From patients to policy: Population intervention effects in epidemiology. *Epidemiology*, *28*(4), 525–528. doi:10.1097/EDE.0000000000000648

Westreich, D., Edwards, J. K., Cole, S. R., Platt, R. W., Mumford, S. L., & Schisterman, E. F. (2015). Imputation approaches for potential outcomes in causal inference. *International Journal of Epidemiology*, *44*(5), 1731–1737. doi:10.1093/ije/dyv135

Westreich, D., Edwards, J. K., Lesko, C. R., Cole, S. R., & Stuart, E. A. (2019). Target validity and the hierarchy of study designs. *American Journal of Epidemiology*, *188*(2), 438–443. doi:10.1093/aje/kwy228

4

Diagnostic Testing, Screening, and Surveillance

Surveillance, diagnostic testing, and screening are central (and related) concepts in epidemiology, and are addressed together in this chapter. Critical concepts covered the following include active and passive surveillance; issues in diagnostic testing including sensitivity, specificity, and positive predictive value (PPV); and screening for disease. We also briefly cover very basic bias, or sensitivity, analysis.

4.1 DESCRIPTION AND PREDICTION

Both description and prediction are important goals of epidemiology and differ in important ways from causal epidemiology (Chapter 3). Here, we will differentiate between them as follows.

4.1.1 Description

Descriptive epidemiology is noncausal analysis which addresses chiefly the observed data, although often researchers wish to use the observed data to describe a broader population. With this definition of description, it may be reasonably argued that no measures of uncertainty are needed outside of those encompassing measurement error. For example, if one is concerned with only the 1,000 members of a study sample, then the number of those individuals who have (for example) active hepatitis C infection at the moment of inquiry is a fixed number, and error is only introduced if hepatitis status is measured imperfectly. However, it is rare that we wish to merely describe the limited number of individuals in front of us: more often we wish to say something about the population from which people were sampled, often at random (or at least with some amount of random error).

Two key places where you can locate descriptive epidemiology are in public health surveillance (which we discuss at length later) and as "Table 1" of many reports in the peer-reviewed literature. In the latter case, Table 1 is typically a description of the characteristics of a study sample, typically collected at study baseline. By baseline we might mean a randomized trial population at time of randomization or the observational cohort at time 0 for follow-up.

Epidemiology by Design: A Causal Approach to the Health Sciences. Daniel Westreich, Oxford University Press (2020). © Oxford University Press.
DOI: 10.1093/oso/9780190665760.001.0001

4.1.2 Prediction

Prediction here will refer to noncausal analysis which uses the observed data to make statements (predictions) beyond the observed data. For example, we might consider *diagnostic testing*, which is often used on individuals reporting symptoms to determine whether individuals have a disease or not in the present moment—this is predictive in the sense that the true disease state is not directly observed. Such work is intimately connected with measurement error and misclassification; as such, it is also closely related to descriptive epidemiology (How can we know how many cases of disease there are if we can't diagnose that disease accurately?) as well as causal epidemiology (How can we assess the effect of an exposure on a disease if one or both is not diagnosed—or measured—accurately?).

Another example of predictive epidemiology is *prognostic testing*, in which we try to predict something about the future course or outcome (the prognosis) of a disease among individuals known to have a disease. Still another example is to characterize which individuals are most likely to benefit from an established public health intervention—variants on this approach are what is often meant by "precision medicine." Indeed, while some define clinical epidemiology as the study of health outcomes (Weiss, 2006), we feel that what makes clinical epidemiology distinct from epidemiology in general is a greater focus on the diagnostic and prognostic models most relevant to clinical care (Porta, 2014).

We have mentioned a few ways in which causal and predictive paradigms may overlap or inform each other, so it is worth noting as well that causal effects are also clearly predictive. For example, if we know that smoking causes lung disease, then knowing that someone is a smoker might well help us diagnose someone with lung disease. But we consider causal epidemiology distinct from prediction in this book. Broadly, in causal approaches, we ask questions about the impact of a specific exposure on a specific outcome. Our ultimate goal is that of intervening on the exposure to reduce negative (or improve positive) health outcomes: that is, our goal is specifically improving health. By contrast in predictive approaches, we may try to identify a population which is likely to experience high rates of an outcome and thus may require increased resources while remaining disinterested in the specific causes of outcomes. Or we may ask questions about exposures, as in diagnostic testing to determine an exposure condition. Thus, while one can view causal inference as a special case of prediction, there is a useful distinction to be made between the two paradigms. (For more on this distinction related to issues of "Big Data," see Box 4.1.)

One final but critical note is that *screening* for disease—a kind of prediction—is distinct from the preceding examples of predictive epidemiology. Unlike diagnostic and prognostic testing, screening is generally discussed as being applied at the population (not individual) level to a presumptively asymptomatic population (Morrison, 1985). Thus screening should be considered a public health approach to a greater degree than is diagnostic or prognostic testing. In fact, screening may be done with the same tests as diagnostic testing, but because screening is done

Box 4.1

Big Data and Epidemiologic Paradigms

Big data are sometimes differentiated from "small" or "regular" data in terms of volume (amount of data), velocity (data come to us in real time/are updated frequently), and/or variety (often less structured, or from less traditional sources such as social media). It has been observed (Mooney et al., 2015) that numerous issues raised by big data are of different magnitude but not different type, including choosing variables for control of confounding (see Chapter 6 for more on what we mean here).

One point that should be raised, however, is that, at this writing, much work in big data—and related, in machine learning, which is often an approach taken to grappling with "big" datasets—has focused on prediction. Websites that want you to buy things—and want to use your purchasing history to try to get you to buy things—do not need to know *why* you are likely to buy a widget, only whether or not you are likely to. As you read accounts of big data in the media, that might be a thing to consider: Are they asking causal questions or predictive ones? And, perhaps, are they asking predictive questions but interpreting the answers as if they are causal? Of note, efforts to use big data (such as electronic health records) for surveillance purposes are ongoing despite some past failures (Lazer & Kennedy, 2015).

---

on asymptomatic ("healthy") individuals, the intent, ethics, and mathematics are distinct and must be clear. We discuss the distinction between screening and diagnostic testing further later.

In the remainder of the chapter, we introduce diagnostic testing, screening, and surveillance and the biases that arise in each and basic strategies for addressing some of those biases. One important note is that we are, for didactic purposes, introducing diagnostic testing, screening, and surveillance in the opposite order of how these processes often occur in the world. Quite frequently, we conduct high-level public health surveillance for a disease; then move on to screening of selected, presymptomatic populations to gain more specific knowledge; and finally use diagnostic testing on individuals as symptoms develop. However, introducing these ideas in reverse order makes (we believe) for cleaner and more intuitive pedagogy.

4.2 DIAGNOSTIC TESTING

Diagnostic testing is the process of determining whether an individual, usually one presenting in a clinical or other setting with symptoms, has a particular condition—an infection, disease state, or disease—with sufficient certainty such that we can take a next action. Of special note in this definition is the word "process," which implies that diagnostic testing is often not a single test (e.g., a single blood test) but rather a *series* of tests through which we make a determination of the next action. Steps of a diagnostic testing process might involve identifying the characteristics of an individual, asking questions about behaviors or exposures, and applying and interpreting laboratory tests. Each stage of the testing should refine (formally or informally) a clinician or public health practitioner's estimate of the probability that an individual has a particular condition—although all stages of such a process may introduce error.

Diagnostic testing is distinct from screening in that screening is the process of categorizing apparently healthy individuals—who do not present with symptoms—into those more likely and those less likely to have a diseases of interest. As with diagnostic testing, screening often involves multiple tests to refine certainty.

4.2.1 Example of Diagnostic Testing as a Process

Consider the following outlined process: suppose that a cost-benefit analysis determines that we should conduct a biopsy to confirm a particular cancer diagnosis when the probability of having the disease rises above 50%—if the probability of the disease is lower than that, the risks of the biopsy outweigh its potential upsides. Based on a patient's complaints, a clinician believes that the person has a 20% chance of having the cancer in question (we might say here that "the pretest probability of cancer is 20%"). While the clinician might be wrong about the probability that the patient has the cancer, nonetheless, at this point, a biopsy is not justifiable because the estimated 20% risk of cancer does not justify the risks of the biopsy.

Suppose further that there is a blood test that is thought to be worth doing if the probability of the cancer is above 10%—and that people who test positive on this blood test have a 60% chance of having cancer, while those who test negative have only a 3% chance of having cancer.

Since the pretest probability of cancer (20%) is greater than the test threshold for the blood test (10%), we would run the blood test. If it was positive, we would estimate that the patient had a 60% chance of having cancer. At this point, we would decide to perform the biopsy. If the blood test was negative, we would estimate the patient had a 3% chance of having the cancer and might recommend no further action (though we could also consider additional noninvasive testing if some existed).

The literature on diagnostic testing is extensive and this example (and section!) is highly simplified (ignoring the role of likelihood ratios, for example). Our main goal is to remind you that *diagnostic testing is a process*.

4.2.2 Sensitivity and Specificity

Causal inference relies on accurate data. So, too, description and prediction rely on accurate assessment of individual characteristics, especially (though not limited to) who has or does not have a disease. Sensitivity and specificity are canonical ways to characterize the accuracy of such assessments.

Consider the classification of disease outcomes and suppose that each individual under study has a true disease state (i.e., each participant either does, or does not, have end stage renal disease). As well, each individual has the rest of a diagnostic test for end stage renal disease. This test result may or may not coincide with the true underlying disease state. We can consider these two factors (true disease state; test result) in a 2 × 2 table (like the one shown in Table 4.1): true disease states are in the columns, and test results are in the rows (although, of course, you are free to rearrange the table as you find it most intuitive). There are four combinations of disease and test state. We label these combinations as follows: those who truly have the disease and who test positive are *true positives* (they are accurately being declared positive for disease); those who truly have the disease and who test negative are *false negatives* (they are being called negative, but incorrectly); those without the disease who test positive are *false positives*, while those without the disease who test negative are *true negatives* (correctly called negative for disease).

From the table shown in Table 4.1 we can describe and indeed calculate both sensitivity and specificity. *Sensitivity* is defined as the ability of a diagnostic test to identify true positives; while *specificity* is defined as the ability of a diagnostic test to identify true negatives. Sensitivity is calculated from the preceding table as the proportion of those actually positive for the disease $(A + C)$ who are identified as positive by the test (A): that is, $A/(A + C)$. Specificity is calculated as the proportion of those actually negative for the disease $(B + D)$ who are identified as negative by the test (D): that is, $D/(B + D)$.

An alternative formulation of these same ideas is possible in terms of the probability of having or not having the disease ($\Pr(Y+)$, and $\Pr(Y-)=1-\Pr(Y+)$), and the probability of testing positive and negative ($\Pr(T+)$, and $\Pr(T-)=1-\Pr(T+)$). In these terms the sensitivity can be stated simply as $P(T+|Y+)$, which is read as "the probability of a positive test given that an individual truly has the disease" (again, the "|" is read as "given"). From Table 4.1, the "given an individual truly has the disease" restricts us to the "Have the disease" column, and the probability is simply $A/(A + C)$. Likewise, specificity can be written as $\Pr(T-|D-)$ which is $D/(B + D)$ from Table 4.1. This formulation is clearer in being explicit about how sensitivity

Table 4.1 RELATION OF TRUE DISEASE STATUS TO TEST STATUS

	Have the disease ($Y+$)	Do not have disease ($Y-$)	Total
Test positive for disease ($T+$)	True positives (A)	False positives (B)	$A + B$
Test negative for disease ($T-$)	False negatives (C)	True negatives (D)	$C + D$
Total	$A + C$	$B + D$	$A + B + C + D$

BOX 4.2

THE "ACCURACY" OF A DIAGNOSTIC TEST

Reports (including media reports) of diagnostic test breakthroughs sometimes comment on their "accuracy," but it is usually unclear what they mean by that word. In context, it sometimes appears to mean the same thing as sensitivity, and other times it seems to be answering the question "how many people are classified correctly?" (where true positives and true negatives are both classified correctly). Again, however, there is variation in what people mean when they speak of "accuracy," and sensitivity and specificity apply to different people entirely (sensitivity applies only to those who are truly disease-positive; specificity only to those who are truly negative). As such, we recommend avoiding this usage (following Morrison, 1985) and being very careful in interpreting published literature that makes claims about "accuracy."

and specificity relate to formal statements of probability and is not dependent on the axes of a 2 × 2 table being oriented in a particular way.

Both sensitivity and specificity are considered to be independent of the prevalence of the disease in the population under study (which in this case is $(A + C)/(A + B + C + D)$—the total number of true cases as a proportion of the total number of people). Perhaps because of this, there is a tendency to assume that sensitivity and specificity can be generalized to other populations. While such assumptions may be reasonable when considering biological assays, they are on less solid ground if our "diagnostic test" is an interview or related to more social characteristics.

Suppose, for example, that our "diagnostic test" for a diagnosis of autism spectrum disorder is a structured interview, but the depth and validity of the interview may vary with who is doing the interview. In such diagnosis-by-interview cases, the depth of the interview—and thus sensitivity and specificity—may be affected by the interviewer's perception of disease prevalence. In such a case, sensitivity and specificity estimated in a clinic specializing in developmental disorders (where prevalence may be higher) might not be valid in other, lower prevalence settings (see Box 4.2).

4.2.3 Scales, Receiver-Operator Characteristic (ROC) Curves

The preceding discussion of sensitivity and specificity imagines that there is one test result and one true disease status, each of which resolves to a simple yes or no answer. But, of course, reality is often more complicated than that. Imagine that we have a survey of four questions, each answered yes or no: each question answered yes earns 1 point, and so all those who complete the survey have a score

Table 4.2 CAGE QUESTIONNAIRE PERFORMANCE

Yes answers	True alcohol dependence	No alcohol dependence	Total
4	53	0	53
3	43	5	48
2	20	20	40
1	12	22	34
0	14	177	191
Total	142	224	366

Data from Mayfield et al. 1974, on performance of the CAGE questionnaire among 366 patients admitted to a hospital Psychiatric Service of the Veterans Administration Hospital, Durham, North Carolina; the gold standard for alcoholism was classification by a social worker based on interview results.

of between 0 and 4 inclusive. We conduct a study to assess whether the scale correlates with some other, gold standard assessment of a condition.

For example, the CAGE questionnaire for problematic alcohol consumption takes this form, where the gold standard was an in-depth interview from a healthcare provider. CAGE was proposed by Ewing and published years later (1984); earlier, in 1974, Mayfield published data comparing the performance of the CAGE questionnaire to the gold standard, finding the results shown in Table 4.2 (Mayfield, McLeod, & Hall, 1974).

Examining Table 4.2, it is immediately obvious that the prevalence of true alcohol dependence as determined by the gold standard measurement rises with points on the scale (from practically nonexistent among those who scored 0 to highly prevalent among those who scored 4). What may be less obvious is how to obtain sensitivity and specificity measures from this scalar table. A simple way forward is to consider possible cut-points. For example, if we cut our scale at ≥ 3 (i.e., we state that anyone with a score of 3 or 4 is "positive," for alcohol dependence by our scale), then we create two categories: scores 0–2 and scores 3–4. We can then collapse the data into a single 2 × 2 table (Table 4.3) and calculate

Table 4.3 DATA SHOWN IN TABLE 4.2, BUT COLLAPSED SUCH THAT ≥ 3 YES ANSWERS IS A TEST-POSITIVE

Yes answers	True alcohol dependence	No alcohol dependence	Total
3–4	96	5	101
0–2	46	219	265
Total	142	224	366

Table 4.4 Sensitivity and specificity under
a range of cutoffs for number of yes answers,
for data shown in Table 4.2

# yes answers indicating alcoholism	Sensitivity	Specificity
≥5	0%	100%
≥4	37%	100%
≥3	68%	98%
≥2	82%	89%
≥1	90%	79%
≥0	100%	0%

Note that the row labeled "≥3" implies the 2 × 2 table shown in Table 4.3.

sensitivity and specificity for the CAGE questionnaire with a cutoff of ≥3: in the, table sensitivity is simply 96/142 = 68%, while the specificity is 219/224 = 98%.

We can choose *any* number as a cutoff for "test positive": 0, 1, 2, 3, 4—or even 5. Notably, choosing 0 as a cutoff is the same as simply stating that all those tested (interviewed) are *positive regardless of score* on the scale; likewise, choosing 5 as a cutoff is the same as stating that all those tested are *negative regardless of score*. As such we will have six possible sensitivity/specificity pairs, as shown in Table 4.4. One way for you to gain intuition about sensitivity and specificity and how they relate to each other is to think carefully about why and how sensitivity decreases as the scale increases from 0 to 5 and why and how specificity decreases.

We show these pairs graphically in Figure 4.1 (solid line); the standard way to do so is to graph (1-Specificity) on the x-axis against Sensitivity on the y-axis, such that the upper left-hand corner of the graph represents a screening test which is perfect with respect to the gold standard. (Figure 4.1 also shows a dotted line representing the operating characteristics of a test comprising simply a series of 50-50 coin flips: heads, test positive; tails, test negative.) This type of figure is known as a *receiver operator characteristic* (ROC) curve, and it is common in diagnostic testing and screening literature.

In general, the ROC curve is used for two purposes: one is to characterize the overall discriminatory power of a scale, which is measured as *area under the ROC curve* (a measure which is equivalent to the c-statistic; F. E. Harrell, Jr., Califf, Pryor, Lee, & Rosati, 1982; F. E. Jr. Harrell, 2001); c is often calculated automatically by statistical software when performing a logistic regression analysis). The second purpose for which ROC curves are sometimes used is to select an "optimal" cutoff point, usually defined as the cutoff point that maximizes the sum of sensitivity and specificity and is thus, generally, the upper left "shoulder" of the ROC curve. In the case of Figure 4.1, that point is the cutoff of ≥3. This approach—which is both typical and problematic—implies strong assumptions about the relative costs of false-positive and false-negative results. (See section 4.2.5.)

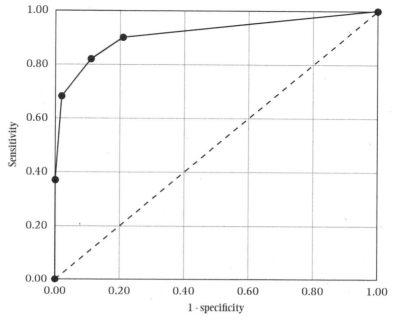

Figure 4.1 Receiver operator characteristic (ROC) curve corresponding to data shown in Table 4.4.

4.2.4 Positive and Negative Predictive Value

Arguably more important than sensitivity and specificity are *positive predictive value* and *negative predictive value*. The PPV is the probability that, given you have tested positive for disease, you actually have the disease—that is, Pr (true positive| tested positive) = $\Pr(Y+ | T+)$, which would be calculated in Table 4.1 as $A/(A + B)$. Negative predictive value is the probability that, given you have tested negative for the disease, you actually do not have the disease—that is, Pr(true negative | tested negative) = $\Pr(Y- | T-)$, which is calculated in Table 4.1 as $D/(C + D)$. For the remainder of this section we will chiefly discuss the PPV as it is far more widely used than the negative predictive value.

Unlike sensitivity and specificity, the positive (and negative) predictive values depend on the prevalence of the disease in the population $\Pr(Y+)$, meaning that PPV is population-specific. The dependence of PPV on the prevalence of disease can be shown if we shift the prevalence of disease while keeping sensitivity and specificity constant. For example, consider Table 4.5, in which sensitivity and specificity are both 90%, calculated in each column as 90/100. Note that this population has a 50% disease prevalence.

We calculate positive predictive power across the "Test positive" row in the same way: among the 100 people who tested positive, 90 of them actually have the disease and so PPV = 90%. Note that this population has a 50% disease prevalence: 100 out of 200 members of this population have the disease of interest.

Table 4.5 EXAMPLE DATA FOR CALCULATION OF POSITIVE
PREDICTIVE VALUE, PART 1

	Have disease	Do not have disease	Total
Test positive	90	10	100
Test negative	10	90	100
Total	100	100	200

Now suppose that true prevalence of disease in the target population of interest was 5% rather than 50% (e.g., for every 50 people who have the disease, 950 people do not), but the sensitivity and specificity remains the same: this is shown in Table 4.6. Sensitivity and specificity can be recalculated from this table as 45/50 and 855/950 respectively: neither has changed.

Now we calculate the positive predictive power across the "Test positive" row as follows: among the now 140 people who tested positive, 45 of them actually have the disease and so PPV = 32%. Which is to say that *even though sensitivity and specificity remained constant, a change in disease prevalence has led to a dramatic change in PPV* (and some change in the negative predictive value as well).

We can derive an alternative formulation of the PPV by understanding that the calculation at hand is (the number of truly positive individuals who test positive) divided by (the total number of individuals who test positive). The number of truly positive individuals who test positive can be calculated as a product of total number of people (N), prevalence of condition under study (p), and Sensitivity (Se), as:

$$True\ positives = Se \times p \times N$$

Total number of positives is *True positives* + *False positives*, where *False positives* can be calculated as a product of total number of people (N), prevalence of not-having-the-condition under study $(1 - p)$, and Specificity (Sp), as:

$$False\ positives = (1 - Sp) \times (1 - p) \times N$$

Thus, we can calculate the PPV as follows:

$$PPV = \frac{True\ positives}{True\ positives + False\ positives}$$

$$PPV = \frac{(Se \times p \times N)}{(Se \times p \times N) + (1 - Sp)(1 - p) \times N}$$

$$PPV = \frac{(Se \times p)}{(Se \times p) + (1 - Sp)(1 - p)} \times \frac{N}{N}$$

$$PPV = \frac{(Se \times p)}{(Se \times p) + (1 - Sp)(1 - p)}$$

Evidently, then, the PPV depends on the prevalence of disease as well as the sensitivity and specificity of the test; the NPV similarly depends on disease prevalence. Reports of PPV or NPV in the scientific literature are *contingent on the prevalence in the study*; such measures should be generalized to other settings (with other measured values of disease prevalence) only cautiously. Better, if PPV is to be reported in a published report, it should be calculated using the disease prevalence from the target population of interest rather than the study sample itself. In many cases, this means that the prevalence of disease must be obtained from some external surveillance source. If there are multiple possible populations of interest, it might be better to report PPV measures over a range of plausible disease prevalence values, rather than only at a single value of prevalence.

Reporting of a PPV based on a misrepresentative study prevalence is a particular danger in reports of diagnostic test accuracy, which often oversample patients who truly have the disease in order to increase statistical power. For example, this is precisely what we show in contrasting Table 4.5 to Table 4.6: in Table 4.5 we showed a study sample with true disease prevalence of 50%, even though the disease prevalence in the target population of interest was only 5% (Table 4.6). Had we assumed that the PPV of 90% from our analysis in Table 4.5 held for the data in Table 4.6 we would have seriously misled readers.

Despite this limitation, positive and negative predictive value are extremely important. If you go into a doctor's office complaining of symptoms and have a diagnostic test performed, how will you interpret a positive test result? The PPV is the critical piece of information that helps you translate that test result into a likelihood that you actually have the disease you were concerned about.

Table 4.6 EXAMPLE DATA FOR CALCULATION OF POSITIVE PREDICTIVE VALUE, PART 2

	Have disease	Do not have disease	Total
Test positive	45	95	140
Test negative	5	855	860
Total	50	950	1,000

4.2.5 Tradeoffs in Sensitivity and Specificity

Earlier we discussed how, for many diagnostic tests, there is a choice between a more sensitive and a more specific test. This leads us to ask: How do you choose? Some questions that point toward the tradeoffs between sensitivity and specificity include the following. In each case, you might want to ask yourself: If I were to answer yes to this question, would that imply that I would want a higher sensitivity or a higher specificity? (Also: can you think of a good example of this?)

Is the disease extremely deadly or contagious if it is missed in an individual? If so, then you might put additional weight on not missing any cases.

Is the next step after a positive test result highly invasive (a biopsy, a surgery) or traumatic (telling a patient they are likely to die within weeks or months)? If so, then you might want to make sure you don't overdiagnose.

Given the disease prevalence in the target population, how much will my choice to favor sensitivity or specificity affect my positive and negative predictive value?

It is easy to see that false positives and false negatives might lead to different levels of harm in a specific situation or for a particular condition—which in turn strongly argues against simply taking the cutoff that maximizes the sum of sensitivity and specificity. A better solution might be some sort of cost-benefit analysis, where the costs of false-positive test results are weighed in some fashion against the costs of false-negative test results for the population under consideration while taking into account the prevalence of the underlying condition for which we are screening. This is almost never done in practice, although that does not mean it is not the right thing to do.

On this last point, "the right thing to do" is worth emphasizing: the choice of sensitivity and specificity—the weighing of the costs of false-positive and false-negative results—is a choice with meaningful ethical dimensions and should (likely) be regarded as a question of medical or research ethics. A related, but larger, point is that epidemiologists often do not see the ethical dimensions of their methodological decisions—and many, many methodological decisions we make as epidemiologists have ethical dimensions to them.

4.2.6 Additional Topics in Diagnostic Testing

A book on clinical epidemiology or screening (which this is not!) will elaborate past these initial points. Here, we note briefly several issues relevant to diagnostic testing, but on which we do not dwell.

Development of clinical score algorithms. There is often a desire among epidemiologists and clinicians to use data to create a clinical scoring algorithm like the CAGE questionnaire for the purposes of improving clinical care as well as health communication and patient education more broadly. Creation of such an algorithm often proceeds by first modeling the data in question using a regression approach (e.g., logistic regression) and then using the coefficients from the regression models (e.g., the odds ratios or log-odds ratios) to construct a score, which is then used as an analog scale for choosing a cutoff. As with CAGE, each cutoff on this scale may have a different sensitivity and specificity. The idea is that a clinician can use a simple checklist to assign a score, which can then be evaluated for risk.

Such approaches are sometimes very valuable. One particularly good example of this is the Atherosclerotic Cardiovascular Disease (ASCVD) risk calculator Goff et al., 2014; www.cvriskcalculator.com], which estimates 10-year risk of heart attack based on age, gender, race, smoking status, blood pressure, cholesterol, and a few other easily obtained measures and which has been used and cited widely.

The c-statistic. The c-statistic is a measure of the discriminatory power of a classifier, where "classifier" is left deliberately ambiguous (and may include a wide range of processes that classify things into two categories). The c-statistic is sometimes regarded as a loose analog of the R-squared statistic popular in linear regression and is addressed in numerous other places: for our purposes, we want only to note that it is equivalent to the area under the ROC curve.

Diagnostic testing with no gold standard. Discussions of sensitivity and specificity rely on the assumption that there is a gold standard for the truth of whether a disease is present or absent. But gold standards are themselves often not quite perfect, and sometimes there is no gold standard at all: for example, we might have two different tests for the presence of a disease, and each test is known to be imperfect for different reasons. This is a tricky situation that can be (and has been) approached in a number of different ways (for example, Miller, 1998).

4.3 SCREENING

As we alluded to earlier, screening is related to diagnostic testing, in that its purpose is to classify people into two groups—likely diseased or likely healthy—often using tests identical to those used in diagnostic testing. The critical difference, however, is that diagnostic testing applies to an individual, usually symptomatic, who has presented to a clinician with some issue to resolve. Screening, on the other hand, is typically thought of as a process applied to people without symptoms.

A complete treatment of screening is beyond our scope; however, we wish to emphasize several points. Because screening applies to the general, apparently healthy population, the intention of screening is quite different from that of diagnostic testing and the process engenders several special considerations, methodologically as well as ethically.

For example, because the process of screening is applied to those without symptoms, we should expect disease prevalence in the screening population to be much lower than in a symptomatic population presenting to a clinician. *Methodologically,* this means that the PPV of a test applied in a screening setting can be expected to be lower—perhaps vastly lower—than if the same test is applied in a diagnostic testing setting. *Ethically,* this means that a false-positive result on a screening test can result in a healthy individual being entered into the healthcare system, which may result in physical and psychological consequences—likewise, if the screening has any side effects, numerous people will be exposed to them (Fletcher & Fletcher, 2005).

More broadly, screening is hard to justify if there is no improvement in health outcomes as a result of it. What this means in particular is that it is only worth screening if intervening in presymptomatic individuals improves outcomes compared to waiting to treat those individuals after symptoms emerge.[1]

An additional point worth considering is the differing perspectives that clinicians and public health organizations put on sensitivity and specificity in screening contexts. Clinicians sometimes prefer high-sensitivity tests: if a test cannot detect disease prior to symptom onset, then it is of low value in control of that disease. Indeed, missing a case of disease in routine screening is sometimes a source of medical malpractice lawsuits. On the other hand, public health organizations (such as the US Preventive Services Task Force) may prefer screening with high specificity because conditions for which we screen are typically quite rare. To understand why, return to our earlier equation for PPV,

$$PPV = \frac{(Se \times p)}{(Se \times p) + (1 - Sp)(1 - p)}$$

From this equation, we note that when p is small, $(1 - p) \gg p$, and so having a high specificity will be of more importance to the PPV than high sensitivity. Considering the data in Table 4.6, in which sensitivity and specificity are both 90%, we would calculate

$$PPV = \frac{(0.9 \times 0.05)}{(0.9 \times 0.05) + (1 - 0.9)(1 - 0.05)} = \frac{0.045}{0.045 + 0.095} = 0.32$$

Now suppose we have the choice between (a) increasing sensitivity to 0.99 and leaving specificity at 0.90 or (b) leaving sensitivity at 0.90 and increasing specificity to 0.99. In case (a), we calculate the PPV as

$$PPV_a = \frac{(0.99 \times 0.05)}{(0.99 \times 0.05) + (1 - 0.9)(1 - 0.05)} = \frac{0.0495}{0.0495 + 0.095} = 0.34$$

which is an improvement over the original PPV. But in the second case, we calculate PPV as

$$PPV_b = \frac{(0.90 \times 0.05)}{(0.90 \times 0.05) + (1 - 0.99)(1 - 0.05)} = \frac{0.045}{0.045 + 0.0095} = 0.83$$

PPV_b, after improving specificity alone, is a vast improvement over both PPV_a (after improving sensitivity alone) or the original PPV. Again, when the prevalence is rare, the PPV is driven by specificity to a greater extent than by sensitivity.

---

1. Of course, one might argue that screening for an infectious disease might help reduce transmission of that disease even if individual outcomes are not improved by early detection.

Moreover, for most real-world screening, the 5% prevalence of disease we propose in Table 4.6 is far too high. Consider cancer screening: true disease prevalence in asymptomatic individuals ranges from 800/100,000 for prostate cancer and 400/100,000 for breast cancer to 50/100,000 for ovarian cancer and 20/100,000 for pancreatic cancer. To put this in perspective, consider a population with a disease prevalence of 100/100,000 (or 0.1%) and a (very good) diagnostic test with sensitivity of 1 (perfect sensitivity) and specificity of 99%. The PPV for this test in this population is a mere 9%; for every 100,000 people screened, the test will find about 100 true positives mixed among about 1,000 false positives.

This result is often seen as counterintuitive. Perfect sensitivity, near-perfect specificity—yet a very low PPV. But such results are typical in public health screening settings, where prevalence of the disease for which we are screening is often extremely low. Again, this leads to serious ethical considerations: those 1,000 people are told (falsely!) that they have a possibly serious health condition and—perhaps—exposed to additional, unnecessary interventions. This may bring with it psychological harm in the form of worry, physical risk if follow-up tests are invasive, and financial risk if they must pay for those follow-up tests. Thus, in screening contexts, public health professionals often care a great deal more about specificity (and, relatedly, overdiagnosis) than sensitivity.

4.3.1 Additional Topics in Screening

As earlier, we briefly address two additional challenges relevant to screening and to understanding the benefits of screening. A book on clinical epidemiology or screening (which this is not) will elaborate past these initial descriptions.

Lead-time bias. Suppose that screening leads to earlier detection of a disease but that earlier detection of disease confers no survival benefit. For example, a new screening procedure detects a certain type of cancer far earlier than existing procedures, but those who are detected with the screen die at the same time as those who were not detected during the screening process. Specifically, suppose we have two people, both of whom develop cancer at age 40 and die of that disease at age 50. Person 1 is screen-detected positive at age 41, while Person 2 is not screened and has cancer detected at age 47. Person 1 is thus followed-up for 9 years, while Person 2 is followed for only 3: however, again, both developed disease and died at the same age, so there is no survival benefit of the early detection.

Lead-time bias is looking at this difference in follow-up time and concluding incorrectly that the difference in follow-up time is attributable to the benefit of the screening itself: that Person 1 lived longer (under observation) due to the screening than Person 1 would have if they had not been screened. To put this another way, lead-time bias is the error of attributing a mortality benefit to screening when in fact screening is simply putting people under observation for longer.

Length-time bias. Suppose you have two types of a particular disease: slow-progressing disease and fast-progressing disease. Diseases that progress more slowly often have longer preclinical periods. Specifically, suppose we have two new people, both of whom become sick at the same time, at the same age of 60.

Person 3 has slow-progressing disease and dies of the disease at age 75. Person 4 has fast-progressing disease and dies of the disease at age 65.

Length-time bias occurs because screening will, over time, tend to pick up more slow-progressing diseases than fast-progressing diseases: in particular, screening when Person 3 is 67 will miss Person 4 entirely, as Person 4 will have died at that point.[2] In such a case, even if screening has no benefits, the people detected by screening may appear to live longer (because they are oversampled by the screening process). This is an example of how selection bias may affect a study examining the impact of screening.

4.4 SURVEILLANCE

Disease surveillance is critical to public health practice: without knowing how many cases of a disease exist, it is difficult to know how to allocate resources to controlling that disease. One useful definition comes from Langmuir (1963), where the author defined surveillance as "the continued watchfulness over the distribution and trends of incidence through the systematic collection, consolidation, and evaluation of morbidity and mortality reports and other relevant data."

Disease surveillance systems take numerous forms and use varied specific (and ever-expanding) technologies but are broadly divided into "active" and "passive" surveillance—categories with fuzzy borders and plenty of overlap. *Active surveillance* describes a situation in which epidemiologists (and others) go out and search for cases of a disease. *Passive surveillance* describes a situation in which epidemiologists let others report cases of disease into a (usually central) collection mechanism.

Active surveillance programs are often initiated by a local or state health department or (in the United States) by the Centers for Disease Control and Prevention (CDC), when the organization in question wants to understand the incidence of a disease in some population. For example, the FoodNet program (presently found at www.cdc.gov/foodnet/) is an active surveillance program founded in 1995 that tracks "trends for infections transmitted commonly through food . . . [it] estimates the number of foodborne illnesses, monitors trends in incidence of specific foodborne illnesses over time, attributes illnesses to specific foods and settings, and disseminates this information" (www.cdc.gov/foodnet, 7 August 2019). FoodNet is a program of the CDC, several state health departments, the US Department of Agriculture, and the US Food and Drug Administration. The program actively contacts clinical laboratories in 10 states to obtain information about infections and, in addition, conducts surveys of both physicians and individuals, as well as population-based studies.

---

2. This is closely related to issues of the prevalence of a disease being a function of both incidence and duration, together; see Chapter 1.

The fact that FoodNet staff reach out to laboratories, clinicians, and individuals makes FoodNet an active surveillance program. In contrast, a passive surveillance program simply lets the data come in, reported by clinicians or others to the center. One example of a passive surveillance system is the Vaccine Adverse Event Reporting System (VAERS, vaers.hhs.gov). Thus, where active surveillance might be thought of as centralized or top-down, passive surveillance is more naturally decentralized, or bottom-up. That said, passive surveillance programs are sometimes legal obligations: in the United States, all states have laws and regulations which mandate reporting of particular infectious diseases to public health authorities, although the list of diseases varies by state. In Massachusetts for example, 105 CMR 300.100 states that

> Cases or suspect cases of the diseases listed as follows shall be reported by household members, physicians and other health care providers . . . immediately, but in no case more than 24 hours after diagnosis or identification, to the board of health in the community where the case is diagnosed or suspect case is identified.

This goes on to list more than three dozen diseases including hepatitis A, B, C, D, and E; smallpox; chickenpox; potential bioterrorism agents such as anthrax; leprosy; and measles (https://www.mass.gov/files/documents/2017/09/11/105cmr300.pdf). Other regulations mandate that laboratories diagnosing certain conditions (including sexually transmitted infections) do the same.

To inform national surveillance, some reportable conditions are also nationally notifiable (e.g., are provided to CDC voluntarily by states). The Council of State and Territorial Epidemiologists (CSTE) makes recommendations annually about which conditions should be nationally notifiable; in 2018, there were more than 120 infectious and noninfectious conditions deemed nationally notifiable (wwwn.cdc.gov/nndss/conditions). In addition, to increase consistency of surveillance across jurisdictions, CSTE maintains a list of case definitions for reportable and nationally notifiable conditions.

Passive surveillance programs are, generally speaking, cheaper to enact than active surveillance systems, but because they rely on numerous individual providers to report diseases, they may not report data as completely as an active system (www.who.int/immunization/monitoring_surveillance/burden/vpd/surveillance_type/passive/en/). Reports from individual providers may likewise be biased if certain providers are more likely than others to report. For example, if providers from public clinics are more likely to report than private providers, then trends in demographics of reported cases may in part reflect the changing demographics of patients seeking care in public clinics rather than all those with infections.

On the other hand, their relative lower cost means that a system relying on passive reporting may draw from a wider array of reporting agents. Whether more complete information from fewer sites (as under active surveillance) or possibly less complete information from more sites (as under passive surveillance) is more useful is a complex decision related to multiple disease- and situation-specific factors.

4.5 BIASES IN DIAGNOSTIC TESTING, SCREENING, AND SURVEILLANCE

As noted previously, surveillance and screening are not primarily about understanding causality. As such, not all of the four systematic errors we discussed in Chapter 3 are applicable here. We discuss these briefly in the following sections (see also Box 4.3).

4.5.1 Confounding Bias

Recall that confounding bias may be expected when, in a directed acyclic graph (DAG), there is an open backdoor path between the exposure and the outcome. In surveillance, diagnostic testing, and screening settings, there is generally speaking no exposure and no causal effect being estimated; therefore, confounding is immediately cognizable as a nonissue. In general, we do not regard confounding as a challenge in predictive modeling contexts: although the cause of scurvy is lack of vitamin C rather than living on a boat, if your main goal is to predict which people are going to wind up suffering from scurvy, starting with the people living on boats is not a terrible way to start. (So long as you don't assume that the risk of scurvy in landlubbers is necessarily zero!)

Box 4.3

Two Fallacies

Robert McNamara was the US Secretary of Defense during the Vietnam War. The *McNamara fallacy* is named for his decision to evaluate the success of the war using what was easy to measure: reported body counts. When we rely only what is easy to measure—say, a so-called "convenience sample" of our data—we can easily introduce selection bias (or related issues) and be misled. See also Basler, M. H., 2009.

The related *streetlight fallacy* takes its name from the old joke of a drunk under a streetlight, on his hands and knees, looking for something. A passer-by asks what the trouble is, and the drunk responds "Lost my keys." The passer-by joins in the hunt. After a while with no success, the passer-by asks the man if he is sure he lost his keys right *here*. "No, no, I lost them over there," says the drunk, pointing deep into the dark field adjoining the sidewalk. "In that case," asks the Samaritan, "why are you searching here?". "Well," says the drunk, "this is where the light is!" Just because you can look for something in the data at hand, doesn't mean the data at hand is the right place to look for it.

Basler, M. H. Utility of the McNamara fallacy. BMJ 2009;339:b3141.

4.5.2 Missing Data and Selection Bias

While selection bias is a kind of nonexchangeability and therefore sometimes considered alongside confounding bias, selection bias may well impact surveillance and screening. If our surveillance program unknowingly oversamples individuals at high risk of the condition of interest, then our surveillance program may mislead us. If our screening program for a very low-prevalence disease relies on a PPV calculated in a setting where prevalence is abnormally high (such as a study that oversampled individuals with the disease), that value may likewise mislead us. The same points hold for missing data: if we are missing data on a sub-sample of individuals in our surveillance program, we may be biased.

Surveillance programs, in particular, sometimes deliberately introduce a controlled selection bias (controlled missing data) in order to gain precision; for example, surveys sometimes oversample minority groups to ensure adequate numbers of responses to estimate effects within those groups. This practice is, of course, fine—so long as those conducting the survey know the denominators of the groups and so can reweight the results of their survey to represent the general population.

4.5.3 Measurement Bias

At some level, missing data and selection bias may be viewed as measurement biases because you are measuring the wrong people or the wrong subset of people. Here, we consider the case in which we are measuring the right people, but with error. The first and perhaps most important point to make here is that our screening discussion—sensitivity and specificity—are the most common ways to discuss measurement bias (especially misclassification error) in the scientific literature. For example, if an outcome is measured with error in a randomized trial (a study design described in depth in Chapter 5), often as not, that error will be described in terms of the diagnostic test characteristics of the test used to determine whether someone has the outcome or not.

The lessons of screening are in fact directly applicable to surveillance as well as causal questions: if your surveillance system relies on a tool that makes errors (every tool makes errors) then the observed prevalence may differ from the true underlying prevalence of the condition under study. In Section 4.6, we give some basic methods for sensitivity analysis and how to proceed in both surveillance and causal (or simply comparative) settings.

Finally, we note that measurement bias is not always a challenge in predictive settings: suppose that (as we believe to be generally true) people tend to under-report the number of sexual partners they have had, and we wish to use reported number of sexual partners to predict risk of having an undiagnosed sexually transmitted infection (e.g., chlamydia). While no doubt the true number of sexual partners is (broadly speaking) a more useful predictor of risk than the reported number of partners, in a clinical situation it is likely impossible for a provider to determine the true number: in reality, the best most providers will be able to do is simply ask their patient a question. Thus, a prediction based on what the patient says—even though it may not be accurate—may be of substantial utility in practice.

4.6 DEALING WITH BIASES: BASIC BIAS ANALYSIS

Bias analysis (more commonly *sensitivity analysis*, sometimes *multiple bias analysis*) is analysis whose purpose is to investigate the degree to which epidemiologic results change with perturbations to analytic assumptions (i.e., how "sensitive" are the results to our assumptions). Note that this use of "sensitivity" is differentiated from the use of sensitivity in diagnostic testing. Vastly more material is available on sensitivity analysis (Lash, Fox, & Fink, 2009; Rothman, Greenland, & Lash, 2008); here, we wish only to provide a simple introduction to some ideas through examples of misclassification.

4.6.1 Simple Sensitivity Analysis for a Prevalence

Suppose we have a condition (say, heart disease) whose true prevalence is 20% and a tool for diagnosing heart disease which has a sensitivity of 80% and a specificity of 90%. The easiest way to proceed is to suppose we have a real population of 1,000 individuals. In Table 4.7, we show the truth in which 200 of the 1,000 total individuals have heart disease.

In Table 4.8, we apply the 80% sensitivity to see that, of the 200 individuals with heart disease, 160 test positive and the remaining 40 test negative (are false negatives); we apply the 90% specificity to see that, of the 800 individuals without heart disease, we correctly identify 720 of them and the remaining 80 are falsely determined to be positive for heart disease. Filling in the right column, then, we find that by using this test we would expect to find 240 cases of heart disease— even though there are only 200 such cases. Our surveillance using this particular test, therefore, would lead us to believe that the true prevalence of heart disease is 240/1000 = 24%, when in fact it is 20%.

That 24% can be calculated in another way, as well. Building off our earlier equations for PPV, we recall that total positives (true and false) can be expressed as:

$$True\ positives + False\ positives = (Se \times p \times N) + (1 - Sp)(1 - p) \times N$$

Table 4.7 RELATION OF TRUE HEART DISEASE STATUS TO TEST
STATUS, PART 1

	Have heart disease	No heart disease	Total
Test positive			
Test negative			
Total	200	800	1,000

Table 4.8 RELATION OF TRUE DISEASE STATUS TO TEST STATUS, PART 2

	Have heart disease	No heart disease	Total
Test positive	160	80	240
Test negative	40	720	760
Total	200	800	1,000

where (as a reminder) p is the true prevalence, N is the total number under study, Se is sensitivity, and Sp is specificity. Observed prevalence (P_{obs}) is simply calculated as total positives divided by total N, or

$$P_{obs} = \frac{(Se \times p \times N) + (1 - Sp)(1 - p) \times N}{N}$$

or simply

$$P_{obs} = (Se \times p) + (1 - Sp)(1 - p)$$

In this case, we substitute in numbers above to find the same result as we found earlier.

$$P_{obs} = (0.8 \times 0.2) + (1 - 0.9)(1 - 0.2) = 0.16 + (0.1)(0.8) = 0.16 + 0.08 = 0.24$$

If we have perfect knowledge of the sensitivity and specificity of the test, however, we can undo this bias by simply solving the above equation for p.

$$p = \frac{P_{obs} + Sp - 1}{Se + Sp - 1}$$

Applying this to the data, we find

$$p = \frac{0.24 + 0.9 - 1}{0.8 + 0.9 - 1} = \frac{0.14}{0.70} = 0.20$$

as expected.

Typically, we do not know the sensitivity and specificity of the diagnostic test being used to estimate prevalence precisely; these numbers almost always have bounds attached to them. In such a case, we can calculate several possible values of prevalence for combinations of sensitivity and specificity which are plausible or consistent with observed values. For example, suppose that we believe that the sensitivity is somewhere between 0.70 and 0.90, while the specificity is somewhere between 0.80 and 1.00. Since, for rare diseases, problems in prevalence estimation are more strongly driven by specificity than sensitivity, we will look at five values of sensitivity (0.70, 0.75, 0.80, 0.85, 0.90) and 21 values of specificity (0.80, 0.81, . . . , 0.99, 1.00).

Thus, starting with an *observed* prevalence of 0.24, the range of possible values of the true prevalence varies as in Figure 4.2, and, given this range of sensitivity and specificity might be as high as 34% or as low as 6%. (Note that the middle of the figure is Sensitivity 80%, Specificity 90%, where the estimated prevalence on the y-axis is 0.20: this is our original finding, see earlier.) This is quite a wide range of possible prevalence; thus, it is essential that sensitivity and specificity be known with as much precision as possible. In this case, note that, for a given value of specificity (one vertical cut through the above figure), the difference in prevalence between a sensitivity of 0.70 and of 0.90 is relatively small, especially at lower specificity; whereas for a given value of sensitivity (i.e., one left-to-right line) the differences in changing specificity by the same amount (0.20) are much more universally large, as much as 25%. For a rare outcome, there are more people without the outcome than with it; thus, a small percentage change in risks of false positives can have a larger numerical impact on the count of positives than a similar change in the risks of false negatives.

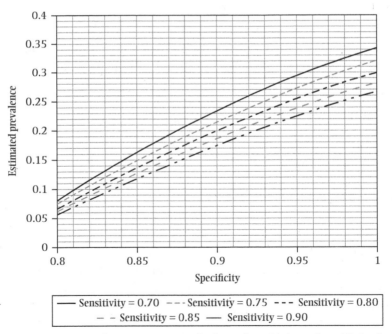

Figure 4.2 Sensitivity analysis over a range of values of sensitivity and specificity for an observed prevalence of 0.24 (and true sensitivity 0.80, specificity 0.90).

Table 4.9 THE BASELINE DATA FOR A 2 × 2 TABLE AMONG 1,000
PARTICIPANTS, 200 OF WHOM HAVE HEART DISEASE AT BASELINE

Baseline exposure	Vital status at end of 10 years		Total
	Dead	Alive	
Have heart disease	.		200
No heart disease			800
Total			1,000

4.6.2 Basic Sensitivity Analysis for a Risk Difference

Now, instead of considering only a single value of prevalence, we consider a risk difference. Suppose we consider heart disease as the exposure, starting with the 1,000 people we saw before but reorienting our 2 × 2 table to put these exposures on the rows, as in Table 4.9. Note that, right now, we are entering the *true*, not misclassified, number of exposed and unexposed individuals into this table.

Suppose these individuals are followed-up for 10 years to see who dies and who does not, resulting in the full 2 × 2 table shown in Table 4.10. The 10-year risk difference from Table 4.10 can be calculated as 50/200 − 120/800, or 10%.

However, now suppose that we were unable to classify exposure correctly, just as in our preceding example, with a sensitivity of 80% and a specificity of 90%. We expect 20% of those who truly have heart disease to be classified as free of heart disease at baseline and 10% of those who truly do not have heart disease to be classified as having heart disease at baseline. As in Table 4.8, we anticipate 40 of the 200 of those in the exposed ("Have heart disease") row to be misclassified into the unexposed row and 80 of those in the unexposed ("No heart disease") row to be misclassified into the exposed row.

Further assuming that such exposure misclassification is *nondifferential* with respect to the outcome—that is, that it operates the same way in those who later developed the outcome as those who did not—then, of the 50 exposed deaths, we expect 10 (20% of 50) to be mistakenly classified as *unexposed deaths*, and, of the 150 exposed alive, we expect 30 (20% of 150) to be mistakenly classified as *unexposed alive*. Similarly, we expect that of the 120 unexposed deaths, 12 (10% of 120) will be mistakenly classified as exposed deaths, and 68 (10%) of the 680 unexposed alive will be mistakenly classified as exposed alive.

Table 4.10 DATA FROM TABLE 4.9, AFTER 10 YEARS OF FOLLOW-
UP TO DETERMINE VITAL STATUS

Baseline exposure	Vital status at end of 10 years		Total
	Dead	Alive	
Have heart disease	50	150	200
No heart disease	120	680	800
Total	170	830	1,000

Thus, in Table 4.11, the number of *exposed deaths* actually equals $50 \times Se + 120 \times (1 - Sp) = 52$, while the number of exposed alive at the end of follow-up equals $150 \times Se + 680 \times (1 - Sp) = 188$. As in Table 4.8, the total number of those who are thought to have heart disease in this setting is $52 + 188 = 240$ (Table 4.8, row total for "Test positive"). Similar calculations yield the entries in the "No heart disease" row.

Now if we calculate the risk difference from the misclassified data in Table 4.11, we get 52/240 − 118/760, or 6.1%. This is biased toward the null; that is, it is closer to the value of the risk difference indicating no difference between groups (which is 0) than is the truth (10% > 6.1% > 0). Bias toward the null is what we expect to find with nondifferential misclassification of the exposure (although chance can show us any sort of bias (Jurek, Greenland, Maldonado, & Church, 2005)). This expectation is because when an imperfect diagnostic test randomly chooses some of those with heart disease and analyzes them as if they have no heart disease, and vice versa, then those who are classified as having heart disease and those without appear *more similar to each other than they really are* (again, only on average). When two groups are more similar to each other, we should expect a contrast measure comparing the two groups (in this case a risk difference) to be closer to the value which indicates that there is no difference between them: hence, the expectation of bias toward the null.

How do we undo this error of misclassification? Earlier, we gave an equation for determining true prevalence in the face of misclassification of the prevalence. Since we have specified that our misclassification is independent of the outcome status, we can use the same procedure here within each outcome. Among the dead, we simply apply the same equation from above $\left(p = \dfrac{p_{obs} + Sp - 1}{Se + Sp - 1} \right)$ where p_{obs} is calculated as 52/170, and find $p = 0.2941$; multiplying that by 170 we find a count of exposed dead of 50 and unexposed dead of 120, just as in the correctly classified data in Table 4.10. Similarly, applying that equation among those alive at end of follow-up (where p_{obs} = 188/830) yields $p = 0.1807$; multiplying that by 830, we find an exposed alive and unexposed alive counts of 150 and 680, again, just as in the correctly classified data in Table 4.10.

If we did *not* know the true value of the sensitivity and specificity with which exposure was classified in Table 4.11, sensitivity analysis could proceed in a similar way to the example for prevalence. Given the observed data under

Table 4.11 DATA FROM TABLE 4.10, AFTER THE MISCLASSIFICATION
DUE TO IMPERFECT SENSITIVITY AND SPECIFICITY

Baseline exposure	Vital status at end of 10 years		Total
	Dead	Alive	
Have heart disease	52	188	240
No heart disease	118	642	760
Total	170	830	1000

Table 4.12 RISK DIFFERENCES FOR DATA
IN TABLE 4.11 UNDER DIFFERENT ASSUMPTIONS
ABOUT TRUE SENSITIVITY AND SPECIFICITY

Sensitivity	Specificity		
	0.8	0.9	1.0
0.7	0.304	0.104	0.071
0.8	0.300	0.100	0.067
0.9	0.297	0.097	0.063

Note that, of course, we know the true sensitivity and specificity (0.8 and 0.9); applying
those yields the true risk difference as calculated
from the correctly classified data of Table 4.10.

misclassification (as in Table 4.11) and for each possible combination of sensitivity (e.g., [0.7, 0.8, 0.9]) and specificity (e.g., [0.8, 0.9, 1.0]) we could calculate
the number of participants in each square of the 2 × 2 table and thus the risk difference for each combination of sensitivity and specificity. The results (though
not the numbers in each 2 × 2 table) are shown in Table 4.12. Of course, the
truth ($Se = 0.8$, $Sp = 0.9$) yields the true risk difference (0.100). Note here, as in
the previous example, estimated risk difference changes radically more across
different assumptions about specificity than across different assumptions about
sensitivity.

Differentially misclassified data poses more complex issues than what we
addressed earlier. Here, we have given you a taste of how we can use sensitivity
and specificity—even imperfect guesses at sensitivity and specificity—to help
clarify simple analyses subject to misclassification bias.

4.7 SUMMARY

In this chapter, we briefly covered aspects of surveillance, diagnostic testing, and
screening, including an introduction to sensitivity and specificity and PPV, as well
as a brief introduction to how those quantities relate to measurement error and
bias analysis for recovery from measurement error.

Surveillance is the foundation of public health action. Surveillance can be active or passive, and each approach has advantages and disadvantages.

Diagnostic testing is testing done in a person with disease symptoms, usually
upon presentation to a clinician. Diagnostic testing can be viewed as a process,
rather than a single test. A single diagnostic test can be characterized in terms
of sensitivity and specificity. Perhaps more useful is PPV, which is a function not
only of the test but also of population prevalence of disease; beware the study that
reports a PPV based on a nonrepresentative disease prevalence!

Public health screening is similar in many ways to diagnostic testing but
differentiated by the key fact that it is applied to presumptively healthy and

symptom-free individuals. Because of this, screening requires us to consider a different set of ethical and mathematical challenges than diagnostic testing.

REFERENCES

Ewing, J. A. (1984). Detecting alcoholism. The CAGE questionnaire. *Journal of the American Medical Association, 252*(14), 1905–1907.

Fletcher, R. W., & Fletcher, S. W. (2005). *Clinical epidemiology: The essentials* (4th ed.). Baltimore: Lippincott Williams & Wilkins.

Goff, D. C. Jr., Lloyd-Jones, D. M., Bennett, G., Coady, S., D'Agostino, R. B., Gibbons, R., . . . Tomaselli, G. F.; American College of Cardiology/American Heart Association Task Force on Practice Guidelines. (2014). 2013 ACC/AHA guideline on the assessment of cardiovascular risk: A report of the American College of Cardiology/American Heart Association Task Force on Practice Guidelines. *Circulation, 129*(25 Suppl 2), S49–73.

Harrell, F. E., Jr., Califf, R. M., Pryor, D. B., Lee, K. L., & Rosati, R. A. (1982). Evaluating the yield of medical tests. *Journal of the American Medical Association, 247*(18), 2543–2546.

Harrell, F. E. J. (2001). *Regression modeling strategies*. New York: Springer-Verlag.

Jurek, A. M., Greenland, S., Maldonado, G., & Church, T. R. (2005). Proper interpretation of non-differential misclassification effects: Expectations vs observations. *International Journal of Epidemiology, 34*(3), 680–687. doi:10.1093/ije/dyi060

Langmuir, A. D. (1963). The surveillance of communicable diseases of national importance. *New England Journal of Medicine, 268*, 182–192.

Lash, T. L., Fox, M. P., & Fink, A. K. (2009). *Applying quantitative bias analysis to epidemiologic data*. New York: Springer.

Lazer, D., & Kennedy, R. (2015). What we can learn from the epic failure of Google Flu Trends. *WIRED*. Retrieved from https://www.wired.com/2015/10/can-learn-epic-failure-google-flu-trends/

Mayfield, D., McLeod, G., & Hall, P. (1974). The CAGE questionnaire: Validation of a new alcoholism screening instrument. *American Journal of Psychiatry, 131*(10), 1121–1123. doi:10.1176/ajp.131.10.1121

Miller, W. C. (1998). Bias in discrepant analysis: When two wrongs don't make a right. *Journal of Clinical Epidemiology, 51*(3), 219–231.

Morrison, A. S. (1985). *Screening in chronic disease*. New York: Oxford University Press.

Porta, M. (Ed.). (2014). *A dictionary of epidemiology* (6th ed.). New York: Oxford University Press.

Rothman, K. J., Greenland, S., & Lash, T. L. (2008). *Modern epidemiology* (3rd ed.). Philadelphia: Lippincott Williams & Wilkins.

Weiss, N. S. (2006). *Clinical epidemiology: The study of the outcome of illness* (3rd ed.). New York: Oxford University Press.

SECTION II

Epidemiology by Design

5

Randomized Trials

A randomized trial is a study in which the investigator *randomly assigns each participant* to receive one of two or more *interventions* and then follows-up those participants for a *set period of time* to examine an outcome—frequently either the *incidence of one or more specified outcomes*, or *changes in measures of an outcome over time*.

Randomized trials are an excellent study design for producing results with high *internal validity*—that is, which accurately estimate causal effects within the group of participants in the study (the study sample). However, randomized trials often have stringent inclusion and exclusion criteria, which means that the people actually included in the study may not represent the people to whom we wish to apply the results (the target population, as defined in Chapter 3). Thus, while randomized trials may produce results with high internal validity, those results may lack *external validity* for many relevant *target populations* (Shadish, Cook, & Campbell, 2002, p. 472; Westreich, Edwards, Lesko, Cole, & Stuart, 2019).

As an example, suppose we wish to understand whether a single dose of a (fictional) newly developed anti-inflammatory vaccine prevents having a first heart attack. A randomized trial could be constructed, for example, by enrolling 1,000 participants who have never had a heart attack, who consent to randomization. For each participant, we flip a coin: heads, the participant is assigned to receive the vaccine; tails, the participant is assigned to receive a placebo injection (i.e., an inactive injection with no biological effects, which is indistinguishable from the vaccine). Ideally, we then follow all 1,000 participants for 5 years, count the number of heart attacks in each group, and compare risk of heart attack between our two groups.

The result of this comparison will be an estimate of the sample average causal effect of our vaccine (compared to placebo) on risk of heart attack, where "sample" here notates that we are estimating the average causal effect within our study sample. This sample average causal effect of the vaccine might be the same as the average causal effect for a particular target population, but if the people in the target population are systematically different (e.g., younger) than those in the trial population, that will not in general be the case.

Epidemiology by Design: A Causal Approach to the Health Sciences. Daniel Westreich, Oxford University Press (2020). © Oxford University Press.
DOI: 10.1093/oso/9780190665760.001.0001

5.1 MECHANICS

The gritty mechanics of actually running a randomized trial are well beyond the scope of this book. However, we will briefly address here some issues in the mechanics of a randomized trial that relate to epidemiologic methods.

5.1.1 Specifying a Study Question

The first challenge in conducting a randomized trial is identifying a combination of treatment (or intervention) and outcomes to study. In laboratory-based research, randomized experiments are a default tool—in part because it is both more practical and more ethical to randomize Agar plates or genetically identical mice than it is to randomize human beings. Thus, in epidemiology and public health, randomized experiments are usually undertaken only after the accumulation of easier to obtain evidence. For example, only after decades of observational research on the effect of male circumcision on HIV acquisition was there a consensus view that randomized trials of male circumcision (among adult men) could be justified, and three major randomized trials were conducted (finding a result which was very much in line with previous meta-analyses of observational evidence; see Chapter 8).

One important takeaway, then, is that the impetus to initiate a randomized trial is a product of social context as well as accumulated evidence to that point—often, a trial is performed when there is sufficient demand for a more authoritative answer to the question of the causal effect of an exposure on an outcome. We describe such a case in Box 5.1. In that same description, we raise the critical note that it is rare for observational studies and the trials which follow the accumulation of such observational evidence to address precisely the same study question, for various reasons.

Regardless of *how* we get to the point of wanting to perform a randomized trial, we must consider: What makes a good study question for a randomized trial? Broadly, randomized trials require specific questions with well-defined interventions that can (ethically and practically) be randomly assigned. In addition, it is usually highly desirable to only perform a trial if you know precisely how you will use (or at least, how you will decide to use) the information that emerges from that trial. If you don't know what you're going to do with the result of your trial, and in what population, it is difficult to justify the risks inherent to experimenting.

One key aspect of specifying a study question is choosing not only the treatment, but the comparison (control) group. While so far in this chapter we have chiefly discussed a placebo control—that is, control with an inactive substitute intervention, such as a sugar pill—there are other options. Frequently new drugs are compared to either "active comparators" (i.e., an active substitute intervention, if one exists) or to "standard of care." In a standard of care comparison, clinicians are instructed to treat patients as they normally would for a particular condition. A critical takeaway here is the understanding that *the choice of control* (placebo,

Box 5.1

Depot Medroxyprogesterone Acetate (DMPA) and HIV Risk

Numerous observational studies showed that users of the hormonal contraceptive DMPA had a higher risk of HIV infection (Polis et al., 2016); however, there were significant flaws in many of those observational studies, among them poor measurement of important confounders (Polis, Westreich, Balkus, Heffron, & Participants, 2013). Concerns about both the quality of the existing evidence and the underlying study question led to the funding of a large-scale randomized trial enrolling nearly 8,000 women (Hofmeyr et al., 2017).

It is of note, however, that this trial asked a slightly different question than many of the observational studies that led to its inception. Many observational studies compared DMPA users to DMPA non-users, where the latter was a heterogeneous category varying somewhat from study to study but usually including substantial numbers of women not using any long-acting contraception at all. The trial instead randomized to three arms, all of which involved highly effective, long-acting contraception. Likewise, some observational studies accounted for condom use subsequent to DMPA initiation—thus implicitly asking about the effects of DMPA that were not mediated by choices about condom use—whereas the main analysis in the randomized trial was specified to address only the effect of initial contraception to which participants were randomized.

The results of the trial (not released at this writing) will be critically important in guiding policy on this topic, but they will not precisely answer the same scientific question which many of the observational studies were attempting to answer. While policy bodies sometimes privilege the results of randomized trials far above the results of observational studies for making policies (see Chapter 9 for a critique of this practice), one reason they might not wish to do so is exactly that the two types of studies often ask somewhat different questions—often due to ethical constraints in terms of what can be randomized. Another example of this phenomenon is related by Hernán et al. (2008).

active comparator, standard of care, nothing at all) *affects the scientific question being asked at a fundamental level.*

5.1.2 Selecting a Target Population

In Chapter 3, we noted that no causal effect is well-defined if a target population (sometimes called a *source population*) is not specified. As such, every randomized trial should clearly specify its target population (even if that target population is "all humans"). This rarely, if ever happens: a quick look at the medical literature as of this writing reveals that most randomized trials are not specific about to which target population the results of the trial are meant to apply. Lack of specification of the target has clear implications for the generalizability of randomized trials, described later; here, we note only that when a target population is *not* specified, one of two target populations is usually implicit: either that the study sample is itself the target population or that the study sample is a simple random sample of the target population.

Both cases are unlikely except in large-scale pragmatic trials setting (Ford & Norrie, 2016; Westreich et al., 2019). In traditional randomized clinical trials (e.g., "we randomized 500 people to receive aspirin or placebo and followed them for 2 years"), the goal of the trial is almost always to create generalized human knowledge,[1] and thus it is clear that inferences are meant to extend to some target population beyond the study sample. That the study sample is a simple random sample of the target population is likewise unlikely. Traditional randomized trials require individual consent, and it is unlikely that such consent is given or refused completely at random.

Most of the time, the target population is not explicitly identified by the study investigators before initiating a trial. It would be to the benefit of science broadly for this to change and for investigators to clearly state the target population to whom they wish to apply their results before initiating a randomized trial.

5.1.3 Obtaining a Study Sample

Once a target population is identified, we must establish inclusion and exclusion criteria for the trial so that enrollment can proceed. Who is eligible for the trial and why? A key tension arises here: on one hand, representativeness of the target population may be desirable to allow easy application of the results to the target population. On the other hand, randomized trials are expensive, and their costs increase with the number of people enrolled; to keep a trial as small as possible but maintain statistical power, it is often desirable to ensure a large number of outcome events. This, in turn, may lead to oversampling individuals at higher than normal risk of the outcome into a study—a course of action leading to a study sample which does *not* represent the target population. Of course, it also true that oversampling certain groups (with known sampling fractions) may in fact be more desirable for reasons of either efficiency or sufficient power to conduct robust group-specific analysis (subgroup analysis, see later discussion).

Other tensions abound as well: since adverse events can lead to early termination of a trial, investigators may wish to enroll participants who have a high probability of the outcome yet a low probability of side effects of the drug or other adverse events. And social pressures and individual beliefs (e.g., that it is too risky to include older people in trials) can lead to study samples in randomized trials which poorly represent target populations, such as historical cardiovascular disease

---

1. Indeed, investigators will sometimes explicitly promise to human subjects review boards that the goal of the study is generalizable knowledge—generalizable, that is, beyond the subjects being studied.

trials in which women comprised only 25% of participants despite experiencing a far greater proportion of outcome events (Lee, Alexander, Hammill, Pasquali, & Peterson, 2001).

The study samples that result from such arcane and sometimes ad hoc processes may bear little resemblance to the target populations we wish to learn about. And this, in turn, may prove to be an issue when interpreting results with respect to that target population. In particular, we may field a trial that has accurate results for the study sample (high internal validity), but the results of which do not generalize well to the desired target population (low external validity). And even if the trial is representative of the target population, it will not likely be representative of all possible target populations (Westreich et al., 2019).

5.1.4 Study Power

Power is the probability that a randomized trial (or other study) will produce a statistically significant result, given there is a real causal effect of the intervention compared to the control. Recall sensitivity and specificity of diagnostic tests in Chapter 4: if you think of a randomized trial (or any study) as a kind of diagnostic test for the presence or absence of a causal effect, the power of the study is equivalent to the sensitivity of that test.

The power of a study is determined by numerous factors. Chief among these is the size of the true causal effect being studied. This is, of course, unknown, but we estimate power using speculative values, hopefully guided by prior knowledge and the published literature (see also Box 5.2). Other factors include the number of participants in each arm of the trial and the number of outcomes expected in each arm. The number of outcomes itself can be regarded as a function of study length and number of participants, as well as baseline risks. Finally, the desired Type I error rate (see later discussion) and the estimated variance of the effect estimate under consideration must be determined.

The *Type I error rate* is typically called *alpha* and is defined as the probability that you make a false-positive error: that is, assuming that there is no difference between risk in two arms of a trial, what is the probability that you falsely conclude that a difference exists? (Going back to the analogy of the randomized trial as a diagnostic test, this quantity is the same as 1 minus the specificity.) The *Type II error rate* (or *beta*) is simply the probability that you make a false-negative error: that is, assuming there is a difference in risk between your two arms, what is the probability that you conclude otherwise (analogous to 1 minus the sensitivity—or, in fact, one minus study *power*). Typically alpha—our acceptable Type I error rate—is set to a low value, most often (and arbitrarily) to 0.05, while beta is likewise set to a low value, such as 20% or 10% (producing high power, of 80% or 90%, respectively). As with screening, there are ethical questions raised by the probability of false-negative and false-positive results from a study, and the ethical implications of Type I and II error levels should be considered when setting those levels.

Box 5.2

P-VALUES AND 95% CONFIDENCE LIMITS

For a two-arm randomized trial, we usually define the "null hypothesis" as "there is no difference between treatment arms being studied."[a] For example, we might hypothesize that the active drug prevents death no better than a placebo. Given this, one definition of a p-value is "the probability that, if the null hypothesis was true (there truly was no difference between trial arms) and all of our assumptions are met, we would see a value of the test statistic this extreme or more extreme by chance alone." The phrase "a value of the test statistic" can be reasonably thought of to mean "differences between the arms of the trial."

In a randomized trial with a clearly prespecified hypothesis being tested (and randomization to give us exchangeability in expectation (see later discussion), as well as assumptions of no measurement error and no losses to follow-up or missing data), the p-value can be used and interpreted straightforwardly (although voices are growing louder in favor of abandoning it altogether; see Amrhein, Greenland, & McShane, 2019). However, in a prospective cohort study (Chapter 6) or another observational setting, the interpretation of the p-value is difficult if not impossible because the existence of systematic error (e.g., confounding) ensures that there are always issues beyond "chance alone." There are numerous papers about the utility of the p-value in epidemiology: some useful references include Poole (2001) and Stang, Poole, and Kuss (2010).

The 95% confidence limits are defined even more confusingly than the p-value: "if we were to repeat this study infinite times, 95% of the 95% confidence intervals would contain the true value of the effect under study." What that interpretation does not say may be more illuminating than what it does: one *incorrect* interpretation is, "there is a 95% chance that the true value falls inside the 95% confidence limits." As with p-values, we can only address this point in passing (Poole, 2001).

---

[a] For a *superiority trial*. In a *noninferiority trial*, the null hypothesis is different.

5.1.5 Create Study Protocols

Early in the process of fielding a randomized trial, the investigator must write the *study protocol*, which describes precisely how the study will be conducted, including subject recruitment and enrolment and informed consent procedures, randomization procedures, analysis plan, a plan for data safety and monitoring, and contingency plans for potential adverse events. Of particular note here is the need to preregister the analysis plan before embarking on data collection (e.g., at clinicaltrials.gov). This step—beyond approval by human subjects review board (see the later discussion on randomized trial ethics)—helps ensure that the main analyses are transparent and that temptations to change analysis plans at the last minute (in hopes of a more impressive result, for example) are checked. A study protocol is typically submitted to the human subject review board as well as to sites like clinicaltrials.gov in the process of getting approval to begin enrolling a trial.

5.1.6 Randomization and Assigning a Treatment

After a study protocol has been approved and subjects are being enrolled into the trial, the question arises about how to actually assign the study treatment or intervention to subjects in a random manner. There are several types of randomization; here, we will describe three approaches briefly: individual randomization, blocked randomization, and cluster randomization. *Individual randomization* is as simple as it sounds: effectively, a doctor flips a fair coin for each patient, assigning one treatment for heads and another for tails. (In practice, such individual randomization often proceeds from a series of sealed envelopes or web-based program rather than a physical coin, but the principle of the coin toss is sound.)

Blocked randomization is a slightly more complicated approach which ensures greater balance in smaller samples: the randomization procedure involves a series of fixed blocks of a set size, such that each block contains equal numbers of each trial arm in a random order. For example, with a block size of four units, with two trial arms A and B, possible AB-balanced blocks are: AABB, ABBA, ABAB, BABA, BAAB, BBAA. Randomization proceeds by selecting one of those six blocks at random, then applying that order to a group of four trial enrollees. Ideally, then another—usually different—block is selected and applied, and so on. Such an approach guarantees that the count of those assigned to A and B will never differ by more than 2—which in a small trial (or well-defined subgroups) may be advantageous. At the same time, choosing a different set of four blocks each time prevents predictable blocks.[2]

Cluster randomization, though it sounds similar to blocked randomization, is an approach in which the individual is not the unit of randomization: rather, groups of individuals, such as communities, villages, or school classrooms, are randomized. In such studies the unit of analysis is typically the cluster rather than the individual, and thus the effective n is much lower than the number of individuals in the study.

5.1.7 Blinding

An essential part of the randomization process is blinding (or *masking*). Blinding is the process in which people involved in the trial deliberately hide information

2. In a real implementation, additional blocks may be released toward the end of randomization, or blocks of varying sizes may be used, to help ensure that the assignment of the last few randomized individuals cannot be guessed.

(or allow information to be hidden) from the participants in the trial and/or from themselves.

A common form of blinding is when investigators do not reveal to trial participants which arm of the trial they are in. The most typical method of achieving such blinding is *placebo-control*, wherein an active treatment (e.g., a low-dose aspirin) is matched by an inactive treatment that is indistinguishable from the real thing (e.g., a sugar pill with the same appearance as the low-dose aspirin). If participants knew they were not on the active agent, they might (for example) drop out of the study at higher rates (and could you blame them?), which could make trial results more difficult to interpret. Such participant blinding is not always possible (either ethically or practically); for example, in a trial comparing a surgical approach to a nonsurgical approach to a health problem, blinding might require invasive but sham surgery—which would present both ethical and practical barriers. Using active comparators or standard of care as the control arm may make this process more or less difficult, depending on specifics.

In addition to blinding the participants, those designing the study may wish to blind the study staff and investigators, such that staff would not know whether a particular participant was receiving the active treatment or the placebo. This type of blinding can help prevent study staff from asking about symptoms or side-effects more deeply in one arm of the trial compared to another, which may be a source of measurement error, and from inadvertently disclosing the trial arm to otherwise-blinded participants. For similar reasons, data analysts may be blinded to ensure that analyses are not (inadvertently or advertently) biased.

Usually, blinding is discussed cumulatively and in the preceding order, such that *single blinding* usually implies that participants alone do not know what treatment they are getting, *double blinding* implies blinding of study staff in addition to blinding of the participants, and *triple blinding* implies double blinding and (for example) also blinding the investigators and data analysts.

Blinding can be compromised at all levels, but perhaps the easiest way that blinding can be compromised is in a placebo-controlled trial in which the active drug has an effect—or a side effect—which is noticeable by the study participant. Study participants who notice (for example) far more headaches may conclude (accurately or not) that they are on an active drug with side effects, and such a realization may affect their adherence to the assigned treatment or behavior more broadly.

5.1.8 Follow-Up of Subjects

As with many aspects of rigorous study conduct, it is critical to begin a trial with a clear and unambiguous plan for follow-up, including a plan for measuring the outcome being studied as well as a plan for measuring ongoing adherence to assigned treatment, if applicable. How follow-up is conducted, of course, varies enormously depending on the outcome in question as well as on treatment- and other population-specific factors.

For example, if treatment is something that must be adhered to over time (a pill taken daily or ongoing behaviors), investigators may want to see subjects more often to assess adherence and factors related to adherence over time. Likewise, if the outcome is something that could be missed or forgotten (a transient condition like pain or ache, or a short-lived infection), then it may be more important to assess outcome frequently. If outcome is something that cannot be easily missed (such as heart attack), this may be less true—but frequent follow-up may still be desirable for other reasons, including increasing our certainty about when a diagnosis occurred. We note in passing that if all we know is that an outcome event occurred within a span of time—for example, between visit T and visit $T +$ 1—researchers will often assume that an event happened at the midpoint in time between the two visits, but technically we face a problem of *interval censoring* and should take more sophisticated and potentially less biased approaches to solving it.

One challenge here is patients becoming *lost to follow-up* such that they disappear (e.g., move away and do not inform the researchers or simply stop attending research visits), and study investigators cannot ascertain their outcome status. While we deal more fully with the problem of patients lost to follow-up later, here we note that if we lack outcome measurement on a subset of our trial participants, we are faced with a missing data problem, which may introduce bias. In some settings, outcomes can still be assessed even among patients who are lost—for example, if the outcome is death and the study is being conducted in a location with excellent vital statistics data, then often vital status can be assessed for patients even if they disappear (if only on a delay). Better, of course, is to avoid loss to follow-up altogether, which researchers try to achieve by such means as providing reimbursement for time and effort, or noncoercive incentives, to come back for future visits or follow-up with phone calls and home visits of participants who stop showing up for their visits.

5.1.9 Analysis of Trials: Conceptual Issues

There are two key paradigms to understand when analyzing data obtained in a randomized trial: the *intention (or intent) to treat (ITT) analysis* and the *compliance-corrected analysis*. The ITT analysis is the more straightforward approach and assesses the effect of *treatment assignment* at baseline, whereas the compliance-corrected analysis (sometimes called "as treated") assesses the effect of *actual treatment received* regardless of assignment and is typically used to make inference about the impact of treatment under perfect compliance (e.g., a drug taken exactly as instructed). The "per protocol" effect is different again.[3]

---

3. Some confusion persists in the literature about "per-protocol" effects and how they differ from compliance-corrected analysis. Often, what a per protocol analysis means in practice is that an analyst will start by (i) cutting off follow-up (i.e., censoring; see later discussion) when individuals become noncompliant with their assigned treatment and then proceed to (ii) analyze without accounting for the fact that people often become nonadherent to their treatment regimens for reasons related to the outcome (i.e., without adjustment for the fact that noncompliance may be highly informative). For more discussion, see Hernán & Hernández-Diaz, 2012).

The critical difference between the two analyses is shown in the causal diagram of Figure 5.1, showing a randomized trial of assignment to daily baby aspirin (vs. no treatment) and its effect on 5-year incidence of heart attack. Note that, in this diagram, we differentiate between *assignment* to daily aspirin (far left node) and *actual aspirin use*. The causal effect of assignment to daily baby aspirin is not confounded: as shown in Figure 5.1, there are no open backdoor paths between assignment and the outcome (see Chapters 3 and 6). This is because treatment assignment is solely determined by a random process such as a coin flip, and we omit a node for the random process by convention. Alternatively, we could view the "assignment" node in the figure as inclusive of the randomization process.

In contrast (again in Figure 5.1), we see that actual daily *use* of aspirin is affected not only by assignment to aspirin, but also by other factors. For example, actually committing to daily aspirin is a lot, and some participants who are randomized to the aspirin arm may not actually take daily aspirin the way we've asked them to—the ones who do may be characterized by a cluster of health-seeking behaviors (nonsmoking, regular exercise) which also act to reduce the risk of heart attack. As well, some of those with strong health-seeking behaviors who were randomized to no aspirin may start taking aspirin during follow-up. Thus, health-seeking behaviors may be a confounder for actual daily aspirin use and risk of heart attack. The overall shape of the diagram in Figure 5.1 may apply to numerous trial situations.

Figure 5.1 helps remind us that trials implicitly contain two main causal questions; indeed, most trials contain far more questions than these, but these are the main two. One is "what is the effect of *treatment assignment* under trial conditions?," the answer to which is estimated with ITT analysis. The other is "what is the effect of *actually taking the treatment as the protocol describes*?," the answer to which is estimated with a compliance-corrected analysis.

It is critical to note that these are fundamentally different questions. Clearly, the answers to these two questions will be the same (or nearly so) in some cases: for example, a randomized trial of two different versions of a single-dose vaccine which is administered immediately post-randomization will in general have very few people who do not adhere to their assigned treatment arm, and so the two analyses are likely to coincide. But quite often they will diverge. Sometimes, to highlight this divergence, we refer to the ITT effect as an estimate of treatment "effectiveness" and the compliance-corrected effect as an estimate of treatment

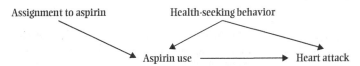

Figure 5.1 A directed acyclic graph for a randomized trial in which participants are assigned to aspirin and followed-up to see if they experience a heart attack, but actual use of aspirin (e.g., compliance with assignment) may depend on other factors—in this case health-seeking behaviors.

"efficacy." The idea is that while effectiveness tells you what treatment actually does in practice, efficacy tells you what it could do, at least in theory.

Numerous approaches can be taken to compliance-corrected analysis. The methods are not complicated for simple cases (a baseline-only treatment, such as a single-dose vaccine) but can require advanced methodology in the case of a trial of, for example, an intervention which requires sustained adherence over time. In both cases, however, the critical point of compliance-corrected analysis is that *treatment actually received is affected by choices and characteristics of study participants*—and as such is an inherently nonrandomized exposure. Fundamentally, compliance-corrected analyses are observational in nature; for example, the treatment a person actually took is not randomized and analysis should proceed by considering the randomized trial as a kind of prospective observational cohort study (Chapter 6) which just so happens to have an initial randomization step. (Although that initial randomization step may be important for analytic purposes.)

Finally, we note that it is common to interpret the effect of treatment assignment, as obtained from an ITT analysis, as an estimate of the effect of actually taking the treatment. This is sometimes the result of confusion over the fact that the two questions are fundamentally different, as we emphasize earlier. But this approach can also be reasonable in that, while the two analyses are asking about different scientific questions, it is nonetheless reasonable to interpret the ITT as a *biased* version of the compliance-corrected analysis. In particular, the ITT is often interpreted as a biased-toward-the-null estimate of the compliance-corrected analysis. The assumption that bias is toward the null comes from the assumption that, in a setting with only one active treatment arm, any cross-over between assigned treatment will tend to make the trial arms more similar and thus act (in expectation) as a form of nondifferential exposure misclassification.

Such a deliberate and carefully stated misinterpretation of the ITT is reasonable when there is only one active treatment arm; less reasonable are questions like "Does the ITT or compliance-corrected analysis have more power to detect a causal effect?" because such a question presupposes the two analyses are asking the same scientific question. Again, they are not.

5.1.10 Randomized Trial Ethics

In the preceding discussion, between creating your study protocols and recruiting participants, you get institutional review board (IRB) approval, which is based on a consideration of the risks to which trial participants will be exposed and the benefits that may accrue out of the study principally in the form of generalizable human knowledge.

One key idea is that of *equipoise*. Equipoise is the notion that it is ethical to conduct a randomized experiment only in the face of genuine uncertainty about whether the intervention is different from the control. Genuine uncertainty does not necessarily mean that investigators believe an intervention has a 50% chance of working, although this is a popular interpretation of equipoise (and is, to some extent, implied by the "equi" part of the word)—and, in fact, it is frequently the case that if you asked investigators to bet on how certain they were that their intervention would have an effect different from that of the placebo (or comparison arm), their wagers would reflect greater than 50% confidence—especially in large-scale randomized trials which are not funded without a solid base of evidence in the first place.

5.2 CAUSAL INFERENCE IN RANDOMIZED TRIALS

Randomized trials are central to the generation of evidence in science and public health, including in epidemiology. However, as we will discuss in more detail later (Chapter 9), typical randomized trials may have good internal validity but poor external validity.

5.2.1 Causal Identification Conditions in Trials

It is often argued that randomized trials are an ideal method for identifying a causal effect. This is true only with regards to (i) causal effects within the study sample (or a target population from which the study sample is a simple random sample) and (ii) for the ITT analysis—that is, the causal effect of the randomly assigned treatment (not necessarily for the causal effect of the actual treatment received). Here, we discuss the causal identification conditions for ITT analyses and consider compliance-corrected analyses in a subsequent section.

Our key causal identification conditions are temporality, exchangeability, consistency/no treatment effect variation, and no measurement error. *Temporality* is met in a randomized trial if we are successful in enrolling individuals free of the outcome at time of randomization. Subtleties may arise if the outcome occurs long before the assigned treatment could have possibly had an effect—for example, a new cancer diagnosis 1 week after ingesting a pill (or placebo) is not likely to have anything to do with the treatment received.

Recall that *exchangeability* can be thought of as "equal risks of the outcome among the treated (exposed) and untreated (unexposed), aside from any effects of the treatment itself." The nature of randomization is that—in expectation (i.e., in a large enough sample)—the average pre-treatment risk of the outcome among those randomized to treatment will be the same as the average pre-treatment risk of the outcome among those randomized to nontreatment. For example, if participants at older age are at higher risk of the outcome than those at younger age, then randomization ensures that, on average, for every 70-year-old randomized to treatment, there is a 70-year-old randomized to nontreatment and the same is true of 20-year-olds. Thus, randomization ensures that exchangeability is met in randomized trials in expectation—though only for the randomly assigned treatment regimen and only at baseline (see Box 5.3). As not all patients may comply fully with their assigned treatment, exchangeability may not hold for treatment

Box 5.3

Differences Between Exchangeability and Confounding

Consider a very small population ($n = 100$), which we are studying for an outcome strongly affected by age (say, outcome is ischemic stroke). If we allowed people to use an intervention or not as they wished—and if older age caused people to use the intervention more readily—we would likely have nonexchangeability due to confounding in our study. (You might want to draw the confounding triangle described here.)

Suppose instead we conducted a randomized trial in this population of that same intervention—and further assume perfect compliance. In such a trial, it would be unremarkable if age was—by chance—not well-balanced between the two arms of the trial because there are only 100 people in the trial. In a larger trial, the law of large numbers guarantees that balance will improve, but in a small trial, we may get unlucky. If we do get unlucky, this would lead in turn to nonexchangeability of the trial arms in that unequal distributions of age means that pre-intervention risk of stroke is not the same in the two trial arms. As a result, our trial might yield an estimated effect quite far from the causal effect of the intervention on the outcome.

This phenomenon—where a strong cause of the outcome is unbalanced between trial arms due to chance—is sometimes called *chance confounding*. This text sharply dissents from this usage. Recall that confounding is defined as a systematic error, and that a systematic error is one which does not go away with increased sample size. Since such "chance confounding" is *exactly* a phenomenon which will disappear with larger sample size, it cannot be confounding. By these definitions, therefore, "chance confounding" is self-contradictory.

Randomization removes *confounding* (the systematic error) entirely but guarantees *exchangeability* (which is partly systematic error and partly random error) only in expectation—and further, only at baseline. We add the important caveat "at baseline" to remind you that selection bias subsequent to randomization (e.g., via lost to follow-up) can introduce nonexchangeability into our study as well.

actually received (e.g., in a compliance-corrected analysis). But for treatment assignment at baseline, randomization on average will balance confounders between arms, *even unknown or unmeasured confounders*.[4]

Consistency is generally met in randomized trials by design: specifically, because patients are given a standardized treatment in a standardized way (either in the same way or using the same protocol), treatment variation is generally thought to be minimal, and so the condition of treatment variation irrelevance is generally

---

4. In addition, if there is a known confounder which remains unbalanced across arms after randomization, you can often improve the precision of your estimate by accounting for that variable in analysis.

met. For example, a vaccine is given by a study staff member or a participant is told to take one pill daily (whether that pill is active drug or placebo) at noon, with a glass of water before eating lunch. Clearly, how (or whether) the patient *actually takes* the assigned pill cannot be enforced under most conditions; thus, there may be meaningful treatment variation for the *effect of the treatment actually received*. Like exchangeability, no (or minimal) treatment variation is broadly ensured in trials for the treatment assignment, though not always for the treatment actually received. Variation in the treatment received will likely increase with the complexity of the treatment itself: treatment with a vaccine is less likely to vary than treatment with a complex behavioral intervention.

Trials do *not* guarantee a lack of *measurement error*. Information bias due to measurement error or misclassification is entirely possible in a trial: for example, if the outcome of a trial is a measured blood level (of LDL cholesterol, say) then it is entirely possible for this biomarker to be measured incorrectly either completely at random or systematically (though, if blinding holds, then hopefully similarly across trial arms). Likewise, if the outcome is death, it is easy to imagine someone being mistakenly classified as still alive when they had actually died or vice versa. By custom, however, randomized trials are usually conducted with very close attention to measurement of treatment assignment and outcome and with close attention given also to actual treatment received (or adherence to treatment) as well as other critical factors.

Recall that *positivity* is the condition that there is a nonzero probability of all study participants getting any possible intervention or treatment. We noted in Chapter 3 that positivity really only arises when considering variables necessary for conditional exchangeability; since a randomized trial provides unconditional exchangeability (i.e., without conditioning on any variables), we meet positivity in a sense by default. But the trial setting gives us an opportunity to dig deeper on positivity: since everyone who enters a trial has *a priori* an equal chance of receiving any treatment under study (because each undergoes the same randomization process), positivity is met in this way as well as by default. In addition, as previously noted, trials only meet unconditional exchangeability *in expectation* and then only in the *ITT analysis*; if conditioning on covariates is necessary to ensure exchangeability for any reason, then we must be concerned with positivity with respect to those variables. That is, if age is unbalanced after randomization and so we control for age in analysis, we must now worry about positivity by age.

It is critical and therefore worth repeating that when studying the effect of actually receiving and/or adhering to assigned treatment—rather than the effect of treatment assignment—these conditions are not necessarily met. This starts to be clearer when we further consider causal directed acyclic graphs (DAGs) for randomized trials.

5.2.2 Causal Directed Acyclic Graphs for Randomized Trials

Consider a group of 60-year-olds who have just suffered a heart attack. We have a newly formulated long-acting beta-blocker, administered as an injection, which

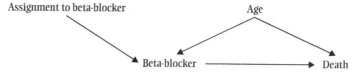

Figure 5.2 A directed acyclic graph for a randomized trial in which participants are assigned to a long-acting beta-blocker or to standard of care treatment and are followed for the outcome of death and in which age influences whether participants comply with treatment assignment.

we wish to compare against standard of care. The outcome of interest is the all-cause mortality over the next month. Broadly, we could proceed in one of two ways: we could enroll participants in a trial which would randomly assign them to either the new treatment or standard of care, or we could allow people to choose which option they want: to opt-in to the new treatment. Suppose further that older participants—who are more likely to die in the next month—are also less likely to choose the new treatment.

Causal diagrams for both scenarios are shown here. In the case of a trial, our causal diagram might look like Figure 5.2. If we performed an observational study, the causal diagram might look more like Figure 5.3. In both cases, we suppose that there is a direct causal effect of age on actual treatment received; the main difference, of course, is that in the trial, the treatment actually received is influenced by the treatment assignment (which is random and so has no arrows entering). In the observational study, the treatment actually received is influenced only by age (assuming the DAG is correct!), with older participants more likely to choose the new treatment.

5.2.3 Causal Inference in Compliance-Corrected Analysis

Given Figure 5.2, if we wish to estimate the effect of beta-blocker use (rather than assignment to beta-blocker) on risk of death, one possible way to proceed is in an observational analysis of the effect of beta blocker use (the node Beta-blocker in the Figure 5.2) on death. In such an analysis, beta-blocker use would not be randomized, and so we would have to closely consider causal identification conditions such as consistency, conditional exchangeability with positivity before interpreting any estimated association as an estimate of causal effect. This

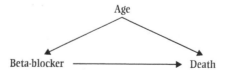

Figure 5.3 A directed acyclic graph for an observational study in which participants choose a long-acting beta-blocker or standard of care and are followed for the outcome of death and in which age influences which exposure is chosen by participants.

amounts to an observational data analysis; we thus defer further discussion of this issue to Chapter 6, where we address the estimation of causal effects in observational data in depth.[5]

5.3 LIMITATIONS OF RANDOMIZED TRIALS

While trials are frequently touted as the gold-standard of evidence (a claim we examine in more detail in Chapter 9), they have limitations that should be addressed.

5.3.1 Not Everything Can Be Randomized

Numerous important health exposures simply cannot be randomized—either for practical reasons or ethical ones. For example, most environmental exposures (especially contaminants such as pesticides, lead, asbestos) cannot be randomized, nor can occupation (and therefore many occupational exposures); exposure to radiation and cigarette smoke cannot be randomized, nor can numerous health conditions whose effects we may wish to evaluate, such as pregnancy and heart attack.

Sometimes we can study the impact of interventions against such harmful exposures—for example, we could feasibly examine the impact of randomization to certain sorts of smoking cessation interventions (and while the ethics of withholding cessation interventions from half of patients may be questionable, they seem clearly less questionable than randomizing participants to initiate smoking in the first place!). But for most conditions listed here and many more, observational epidemiologic research is the main method for studying the causal effects of these exposures.

5.3.2 Noncompliance

In the late 1980s, the (quite possibly apocryphal) story goes, a trial of the first antiretroviral drug for HIV (zidovudine) was ongoing in San Francisco. Zidovudine was not on the market, and so researchers felt confident that while those randomized to zidovudine might or might not adhere perfectly to their assigned treatment regimens, those assigned to placebo could be relied upon to stick to placebo. After all, zidovudine was not on the market yet—how could placebo users get access to the drug even if they wanted to? It is said that a large group of trial participants got together and mixed all of their study pills together—active drugs and identical-looking sugar pills alike—and then took back as many pills as they put in. On average, then, each participant at that party, regardless of their original trial arm, received about half active pills and half placebos—and so received some benefit.

---

5. We could also consider conducting an instrumental variable analysis in this case using assignment to beta-blocker as the instrument. See Chapter 8 for some details.

Strangely (not at all strangely), patients do not always do what they are asked to—even in a trial setting. Those assigned to an active arm of a trial might not adhere to their assigned intervention; those assigned to a placebo arm might somehow (as in the preceding story) get access to components of the active intervention. Such a situation can introduce substantial measurement error into a study.

5.3.3 Loss (Lost) to Follow-Up

Trial participants may disappear from follow-up during the course of a trial: for example, they do not show up for a scheduled study visit and cannot be traced or found. Clearly, participants who become *lost to follow-up* (LTFU) provide no further information on compliance, and we may in addition not record their outcome information at the end of the trial. This results in a form of missing outcome data which will introduce bias into the analysis if there is a relationship between incidence of the outcome and becoming lost: the most common case being that a participant has died and is thus not able to attend a study visit nor be found. If the outcome is death, such bias can be avoided in a setting where all deaths are recorded by a death registry.

Analysis in the presence of LTFU can proceed in several ways: most simply, we can analyze only individuals who are not LTFU, a "complete case analysis" approach to missing outcome data, as described in Chapter 3. Chapter 3 also describes in outline more sophisticated approaches: if we are willing to assume that LTFU can be explained by observed variables (e.g., self-reported sex and age entirely explains who is lost to follow-up and who is not), then we can use missing data techniques such as multiple imputation to fill in missing values or use inverse probability of missingness weights to allow those participants who are not missing to "stand in" for those who are.

Of course, the best (though not always easiest) approach to dealing with LTFU is to not have it: if study participants are willing to give you a contact number, an email address, a home address, and perhaps even a backup contact (e.g., a spouse or other relative), then you may be able to track them down even if they fail to return to the study. In addition, it may be wise to collect data about why participants become lost to follow-up to help inform the missing data methods mentioned earlier.

5.3.4 Adverse Events and Trials Safety

In the course of follow-up, trial participants may experience serious adverse events related to the trial intervention (e.g., side effects of a new drug, such as a serious rash) or otherwise (e.g., an accident apparently unrelated to the study). When such adverse events occur, they must be reported to supervisory bodies, generally including the governing human subjects research board and the Data and Safety Monitoring Board (DSMB) for the study. Such supervisory bodies have the power to halt the study early and may do so if there are too many side effects being reported.

The DSMB is worth describing in more detail: the DSMB typically serves as an advisory body to the funding agency, independent of the study team, and meets regularly throughout the conduct of the study to review progress and reports of adverse events. In addition to halting the study early if the intervention appears to put participants at risk, the DSMB can halt the study early for other reasons: particularly, if study results are sufficiently definitive before the official end of the study that conclusions about the effect (or lack of effect) of the intervention can be drawn. There is a substantial biostatistics literature on setting early stopping rules in clinical trials, so we do not dwell on the particulars here, though we do note that stopping rules must account for the possibility of multiple comparisons. Comparing outcomes multiple times over follow-up, and not just at a single prespecified time point, increases the risks of obtaining a false-positive result.

5.3.5 Trial Generalizability and Transportability

We noted in Chapter 3 that no causal effect is complete if it does not specify a target population, but—again—randomized trials rarely specify the target population to which they are meant to apply. When a trial does not specify the target population, it is often implied that the target population is something along the lines of "the larger population, defined by inclusion and exclusion criteria of the trial, from which the trial population was enrolled essentially at random." This is rarely true, however, in that randomized trials very frequently oversample individuals at high risk of the outcome compared to the true target populations of interest: for example, HIV vaccine trials generally do not enroll individuals in long-term monogamous relationships as those individuals are at very low risk of acquiring HIV, but concentrate instead on enrolling individuals with high numbers of new partners or who report higher risk activities such as needle sharing or unprotected sexual intercourse. As frequently, trials (new drug trials, for example) will enroll participants who are at particularly low risk of potential side effects due to their lack of comorbidities. A full treatment of generalizability of randomized trials and observational studies is beyond the scope of this book, but we discuss further issues in Chapter 9.

5.3.6 Trial Scale-Up and Population Intervention Impact

In addition to the point about trial generalizability made earlier, another key reason that the result of a randomized trial may not scale up perfectly to real-world settings is the gap between idealized conditions of the trial and the reality of implementation. For example, placebos and blinding are generally not an option in the real world, and so causal comparisons from placebo-controlled trials are not necessarily representative of real-world conditions. It is well known that people may act differently when they are being watched: indeed, public health strategies such as directly observed therapy are based on this very idea. Due to this *Hawthorne effect*, the results from a closely watched trial population may mislead us about what will happen when an intervention is moved into a much less closely watched general population. One final concern is if there are spillover (interference) effects of an intervention, as we might expect in a vaccine trial, then this might not be observed in a trial but only after scale-up. Again, we expand on some of these ideas in Chapter 9.

5.3.7 Additional Limitations

Several other limitations are worth noting at least briefly. First, trials require prospective data collection: if a scientific question is extremely pressing, then questions about the quality of evidence may be less important than the speed at which some evidence can be found—for example, from previously collected but nonrandomized sources. Another issue is that the reality of trials funding means that trials are often limited to studying outcomes over shorter periods of time (e.g., 5 years or less); trials therefore typically lack the ability of prospective cohort studies to study outcomes over 20–30 years and, as a result, sometimes rely on surrogate outcomes. Relatedly, trials are expensive and can run into problems finding enough individuals to enroll when outcomes are very rare.

5.4 ANALYSIS OF DATA FROM RANDOMIZED TRIALS

First, we briefly discuss the steps that a formal trial will typically take before analysis (either after the trial has finished or in the midst of the trial as an interim analysis). After final data are entered and data quality checks have been completed, the database is typically frozen—allowing no further changes to the database for analysis. Then the prespecified analyses are conducted, often by a statistician blinded to group identities (see Box 5.4). With results in hand, the trial arms are unblinded, allowing interpretation of the final results. Here, we chiefly focus on ITT analysis; compliance-corrected analysis is effectively an observational data analysis and readers should refer to Chapter 6 for an introduction to methods for observational data analysis.

BOX 5.4

DOUBLE-BLIND CLOAK AND DAGGERS

Occasionally—rarely—this process takes on an element of cloak-and-dagger drama, especially when the trial in question may determine whether a pharmacological agent or vaccine may move toward market (and thus affect the stock price of the company that developed it). One colleague recounts a trial he worked on in which he registered in a hotel under a false name and was sequestered for several days!

5.4.1 Intention-to-Treat Analysis and Beyond

ITT analysis is straightforward: we analyze the impact of assignment to one treatment arm or another on the outcome. Because the causal identification conditions are generally met for the ITT analysis of a randomized trial, crude (unadjusted) analysis of the data is sufficient to estimate causal effects. In particular, analysis from a 2 × 2 table will produce an unbiased estimate of effect in many cases. Similarly, comparing the survival curves for the treated and untreated groups can give us an estimate of causal effect. We can obtain confidence intervals for comparisons such as risk differences in numerous ways, including formulas and nonparametric bootstraps.

As has been often repeated, ITT analysis considers the impact *not* of actual receipt of the treatment, but rather of *assignment* to that treatment. Such analysis proceeds, therefore, *regardless of how well patients adhered to their assigned treatment.* Complications in interpretation of utility of such analysis may arise if outcomes are measured poorly or are not measured in a subset of trial participants (Powney, Williamson, Kirkham, & Kolamunnage-Dona, 2014): various techniques exist for dealing with missing outcome data in clinical trials and elsewhere, though these are largely outside the scope of this work (Little & Rubin, 2002).

We illustrate with a series of simple examples: consider two drugs tested against each other, A and B. We randomize 100 people, 50 per group. In group A, by the end of follow-up (a fixed period of time, say 1 year), there are 10 events (bad outcomes). In group B, by the end of follow-up, there are 5 events. What is the risk in group A? The risk in group B? Risk differences and ratios may be easily calculated from these data, shown in Table 5.1.

Now consider a more complex case, with the same A/B comparison. We still randomize 100 people, 50 per group. In group A, by the end of follow-up, there are 10 events, and 10 people have left the study and are considered lost to follow-up. In group B, by the end of follow-up, there are 5 events, and 30 people have become lost to follow-up. ITT analysis must decide how to count these losses: are they bad outcomes (e.g., disease events), or are they missing outcomes? If the former, we risk diluting effect estimates by effectively broadening the definition of our outcome; if the latter, then how do we decide what outcomes those individuals would have had if (counter to fact) they had not been missing?

As we have discussed previously, risks (and rates, and odds) are reductive measures compared to the survival curves: frequently we want to describe and compare survival curves directly. We discussed some basics of how to calculate (and

Table 5.1 A 2 × 2 TABLE FOR A RANDOMIZED TRIAL OF DRUG A COMPARED
TO DRUG B, RESULTS AFTER 1 YEAR OF FOLLOW-UP

Assignment	Outcome		Total	Risk	Risk difference	Risk ratio
	Yes	No				
A	10	40	50	20%	10%	2.0
B	5	45	50	10%		

draw) survival curves in Chapter 1; if everyone stays in our study until its end (e.g., no one is lost to follow-up; no one has their follow-up time cut off before trial's end—that is, censored; see later discussion), then we can simply apply those methods to each arm of the trial individually and compare the survival curves by treatment assignment (by a method such as the log-rank test; see later discussion).

In real-world randomized trials, some amount of loss to follow-up is inevitable: people drop out of randomized trials for all sorts of reasons. To analyze survival data when we do not have complete follow-up for all participants, we typically assume that all participants who drop out of a study would, if followed for long enough, experience the event being studied—and that our best guess at *when* they would experience the event is given by what we observe from other participants in the study. Later, we introduce the life table method for drawing survival curves in tabled (grouped) data with censoring due to drop-out. We also briefly introduce the Kaplan-Meier method for similar situations and introduce the log-rank test. Throughout the following sections, we assume that drop-out from the trial is an entirely random process, unrelated in all ways to both the exposure and outcome under study; if this is not true, more advanced methods are needed.

5.4.2 Survival Curves With Drop-Out: The Life Table Method

The life table method is most useful when we have grouped data. For example, consider the data in Table 5.2. We show five time points (e.g., each a year apart) including baseline (time $t = 0$), the count of total number n of participants at time t, the conditional survival and cumulative survival at time t, and the number of deaths (d) and drop-outs (c, for censored) between times t and $t + 1$. The conditional survival at time $t + 1$ (sc_{t+1}) is the probability that, given you were alive at time t, you survived to time $t + 1$; in this table only it is defined as $(n_t - d_t)/n_t$ using the notation defined in the header of Table 5.2. By definition, $sc_0 = 1$. The cumulative survival at time $t + 1$ (s_{t+1}) is the probability that, given you were alive at $t = 0$,

Table 5.2 CONDITIONAL AND CUMULATIVE SURVIVAL AMONG 10,000 PARTICIPANTS WITH NO DROP-OUT

Time (t)	n_t	Events between t and t + 1		Survival at t + 1	
		Deaths (d_t)	Drop-outs (c_t)	Conditional (sc_{t+1})	Cumulative (s_{t+1})
0 (Baseline)	10,000	1,600	0	0.840	0.84
1	8,400	700	0	0.917	0.77
2	7,700	800	0	0.896	0.69
3	6,900	600	0	0.913	0.63
4	6,300				

you will survive to time $t + 1$; we calculate this as the product of the conditional survival to $t + 1$ as

$$s_{t+1} = \prod_{k=0}^{t+1} sc_k.$$

Thus, reading across the first row, at baseline ($t = 0$) there were 10,000 participants; $d_0 = 1,600$ of those participants died and $c_0 = 0$ dropped out before $t = 1$, and so conditional survival by time $t + 1$ (i.e., by $t = 1$) is calculated as $(10,000 - 1,600)/10,000 = 0.84$. Cumulative survival by time 1 is calculated as $s_1 = \prod_{k=0}^{1} sc_k = sc_0 \times sc_1 = 1.0 * 0.84 = 0.84$. Similarly, reading across the second row, at $t = 1$, there are 8,400 people alive (calculated from information at $t = 0$, as $10,000 - 1,600$), by time $t = 2$ there are $d_1 = 700$ deaths and $c_1 = 0$ drop outs. Conditional survival in this table can be calculated as $(8,400 - 700)/8,400 = 0.917$. Cumulative survival by time 2 is calculated as $s_2 = \prod_{k=0}^{2} sc_k = sc_0 \times sc_1 \times sc_2 = 1.0 \times 0.84 \times 0.917 = 0.7703$ (and, had we not rounded 0.917, would in fact be *exactly* equal to 0.77). And so on: $s_4 = 1.0 \times 0.84 \times 0.917 \times 0.896 \times 0.913 = 0.63$.

Note that there is a convenient shortcut in this particular table: which is that the $s_4 = 0.63$ is exactly equal to the ratio of 6,300/10,000, or n_4/n_0—that is, simply the percentage of the original cohort still surviving at $t = 4$. This feels intuitively correct—of course that is what cumulative survival means—but this intuition only works in the absence of drop-outs, the fact that $c_t = 0$ in Table 5.2 for all t. Now consider Table 5.3 for a similar dataset but with substantial drop-out. Note that n_t is dramatically lower due to drop-outs.

It is immediately clear that our conditional and cumulative survival estimates may be more difficult to calculate. Here, 2,500 participants dropped out between time 0 and 1 ($c_0 = 2,500$): how should they be counted in our survival analysis? One obvious way to proceed is to first assume that drop-out was unrelated to occurrence or risk of outcome, and thus drop-outs occur uniformly between times 0 and 1. One approach to estimate survival under such an assumption is to adjust sample size for drop-out and use that adjusted (or effective) sample size in

Table 5.3 ADDING DROP-OUT TO DATA PRESENTED IN TABLE 5.2. HOW MIGHT WE CALCULATE CONDITIONAL AND CUMULATIVE SURVIVAL?

Time (t)	n_t	# events between t and t + 1		Survival at t + 1	
		Deaths (d_t)	Drop-outs (c_t)	Conditional (sc_{t+1})	Cumulative (s_{t+1})
0 (Baseline)	10,000	1,600	2,500		
1	5,900	700	200	**?**	
2	5,000	800	200		
3	4,000	600	300		
4	3,100				

calculations of sc_t. Here, we define an effective sample size as $e_t = n_t - c_t/2$; in row 1, effective sample size would be $10,000 - 2,500/2 = 8,750$. We then use 8,750 instead of 10,000 to calculate $sc_{t+1} = (e_t - d_t)/e_t = (8,750 - 1,600)/8,750 = 0.817$. The full life table approach (incorporating the preceding equations) is therefore

$$s_{t+1} = \prod_{k=0}^{t+1} \frac{\left(n_t - \dfrac{c_t}{2}\right) - d_t}{\left(n_t - \dfrac{c_t}{2}\right)}.$$

Now we calculate the cumulative survival at each time point exactly as in Table 5.2, as the product of the accumulated values of sc_t. Because there is appreciable drop-out in this setting, the simpler approach to calculating cumulative survival (e.g., at $t = 4$, $3,100/10,000$) gives the wrong answer for estimated cumulative survival ($s_4 = 0.508$). We show the survival curve estimated in Table 5.4 in Figure 5.4.

The life table approach to survival data is most useful when data are—like these data—grouped into table cells. Alternatives are possible. In this example, we could have assumed that, rather than drop-outs happening over the whole time period, they all happened at the end of each period (after all events). If we make this assumption, then we can calculate survival in each time period as in Table 5.2 using the n at the start of the time period rather than the effective sample sizes; but the sample sizes at each time point would be affected by the censoring similar to what we see in Table 5.4. This approach—assuming that censoring happens after all the events—is similar to the way the Kaplan-Meier estimator approaches survival data and is shown in Figure 5.5. In general, Kaplan-Meier approaches are shown as a step-function rather than the straight line of a life table, to indicate that there are discrete time points at which sample size drops.

Table 5.4 ADDING CALCULATIONS OF EFFECTIVE N_t, AND CONDITIONAL AND CUMULATIVE SURVIVAL TO TABLE 5.3

Time (t)	n_t	# events between t and t + 1		Effective n_t (e_t)	Survival at t + 1	
		Deaths (d_t)	Drop-outs (c_t)		Conditional (sc_{t+1})	Cumulative (s_{t+1})
0 (Baseline)	10,000	1,600	2,500	8,750	0.817	0.817
1	5,900	700	200	5,800	0.879	0.719
2	5,000	800	200	4,900	0.837	0.601
3	4,000	600	300	3,850	0.844	0.508
4	3,100					

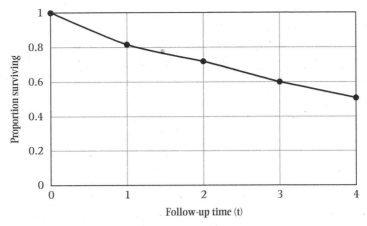

Figure 5.4 Survival curve calculated in Table 5.4.

5.4.3 Kaplan-Meier for Individual Survival Data

As we noted, Figure 5.5 represents a tabled approximation of the Kaplan-Meier approach; the formal Kaplan-Meier estimator is applied in individual, rather than tabled or grouped, data (Kaplan & Meier, 1958; Bland & Altman, 1998). In a trial, we generally have individual survival times—we would generally know that participant 1 died on day 317, not merely that they died between baseline and the end of the first year of follow-up. Thus, we would be presented with data which was a listing as follows: for each person, their total follow-up time, whether they had the event or dropped-out at that time, or whether they were followed-up without event or drop-out through the end of the trial period. We would then apply the Kaplan-Meier estimator to these individual data by treatment group.

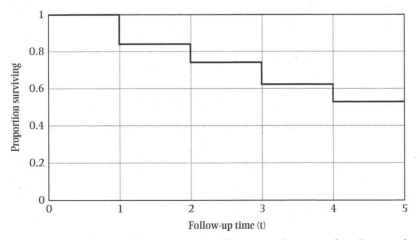

Figure 5.5 A survival curve that assumes that all censoring happens after all events for each discrete time period.

Table 5.5 SURVIVAL FOR 15 UNEXPOSED AND 15 EXPOSED INDIVIDUALS

Person	Day	Exposed	Died?	Person	Day	Exposed	Died?
1	116	0	1	16	197	1	0
2	62	0	0	17	228	1	1
3	110	0	0	18	126	1	1
4	106	0	1	19	59	1	1
5	40	0	1	20	264	1	0
6	260	0	0	21	153	1	1
7	347	0	1	22	364	1	0
8	142	0	0	23	268	1	1
9	233	0	1	24	235	1	1
10	65	0	0	25	233	1	0
11	101	0	0	26	22	1	1
12	346	0	0	27	201	1	1
13	331	0	0	28	183	1	0
14	278	0	0	29	308	1	0
15	317	0	1	30	8	1	1

In Table 5.5, we show the individual-level survival times (in days) for 30 people. The first (and fifth) column lists the person by number, the second (and sixth) column their follow-up time, the third (and seventh) column their exposure status, and the fourth (and eighth) column indicates whether at the indicated time the person died (1) or exited the study either through drop-out or study completion (0). For the moment, we consider only the left side of the table for those who had exposure = 0 (unexposed).

In Table 5.6, we show the same data but ordered by length of follow-up within each exposure group.

In Figure 5.6, we show line diagrams for the survival data in Table 5.6. Person 5 is unexposed and so shown in the left panel (white bar); their line extends to day 40, at which point they die (indicated by a ●). Person 28 is exposed and so shown in the right panel (black bar); their line extends to day 183, at which point they drop out (indicated by a lack of ●).

Now we can apply the Kaplan-Meier formula to these data. The formula for the Kaplan-Meier estimator *within each level of the exposure* is

$$s_t = \prod_{k \le t} 1 - \frac{d_k}{n_k}$$

n_k indicates the number at risk at time k, and d_k indicates the number of deaths (or events) at time k.

We show the calculations in Table 5.7 for a few rows of data from Table 5.6. On day 1, no one dies and no one drops out; there are 15 people at risk; risk of death is 0 and survival is 100%. The same is true every day until the beginning of day

Table 5.6 SURVIVAL FOR 15 UNEXPOSED AND 15 EXPOSED INDIVIDUALS, ORDERED
BY LENGTH OF FOLLOW-UP WITHIN EACH GROUP

Person	Day	Exposed	Died?	Person	Day	Exposed	Died?
5	40	0	1	30	8	1	1
2	62	0	0	26	22	1	1
10	65	0	0	19	59	1	1
11	101	0	0	18	126	1	1
4	106	0	1	21	153	1	1
3	110	0	0	28	183	1	0
1	116	0	1	16	197	1	0
8	142	0	0	27	201	1	1
9	233	0	1	17	228	1	1
6	260	0	0	25	233	1	0
14	278	0	0	24	235	1	1
15	317	0	1	20	264	1	0
13	331	0	0	23	268	1	1
12	346	0	0	29	308	1	0
7	347	0	1	22	364	1	0

40: at the start of day 40, there are 15 people alive; Person 5 dies during the day. The estimated probability of death conditional on those who were alive and in the study (15 individuals) on day 40 is therefore 1/15, and survival conditional on being alive at the beginning of this day 40 is 14/15. Cumulative survival is therefore calculated as $1 \times 1 \times 1 \cdots \times 14/15 = 14/15$.

On days 41–61 no one dies and no one drops out, so the conditional survival each day is 1, and cumulative survival on any of those days remains at 14/15. (At this point, it should be clear that on days when nothing happens to anyone in the cohort, nothing changes in s_t because we are multiplying by $1 - d/n = 1$.) On day 62, Person 2 drops out ($d = 0$). The probability of death on that day is likewise 0, the conditional survival likewise 1, and so the cumulative survival is likewise

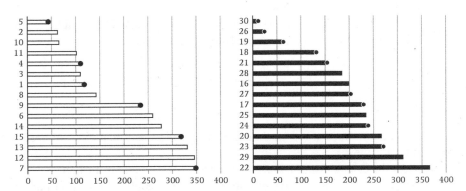

Figure 5.6 Line diagram of the data in Figure 5.6. Circles (●) indicate deaths.

Table 5.7 CALCULATION OF KAPLAN-MEIER SURVIVAL PROBABILITIES FROM SOME
DATA IN TABLE 5.6

Person	Day	Exposed	Died?	n	d	d/n	1 – d/n	s(t)
5	40	0	1	15	1	1/15	14/15	0.933
2	62	0	0	14	0	0/14	1	0.933
10	65	0	0	13	0	0/13	1	0.933
11	101	0	0	12	0	0/12	1	0.933
4	106	0	1	11	1	1/11	10/11	0.848
3	110	0	0	10	0	0/10	1	0.848

1—but *n* drops by 1. The same happens at time 65 and 101 due to drop-outs of
Persons 10 and 11. At time 106, however, Person 4 dies: since there were 11 people
at risk at the start of day 106, and one death, $d/n = 1/11$, and the current survival
(0.933) is multiplied by 10/11, for a total cumulative survival of 0.848.

We can apply a similar approach to the exposed individuals in the table and
then display the resulting survival curves for both the exposed and unexposed
individuals. This is shown in Figure 5.7; note that, in contrast to Figure 5.5, we
here show the survival curve as a step-function because in individual data with
exact times of events, the survival curve does not change as a smooth function.

Once we have applied the Kaplan-Meier method here to draw survival curves,
we can compare the two survival curves in a variety of ways, including the log-
rank test and the Wilcoxon rank-sum test. Such statistical tests have various
advantages and disadvantages, but a discussion of these different approaches is
beyond our current scope (Allison, 2010).

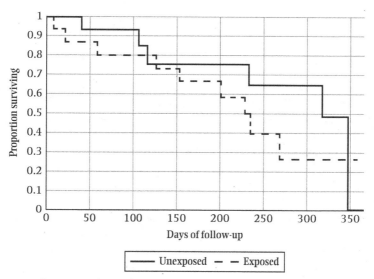

Figure 5.7 Kaplan-Meier curves for the data shown in Table 5.6.

5.5 ADDITIONAL ANALYTIC ISSUES

Here, we explain several more advanced methodological issues in trials analysis. There are two main variations on a standard trial design that we wish to discuss here: subgroup analysis and factorial trials.

5.5.1 Subgroup Analysis

In a typical randomized trial of a single intervention, we conduct a subgroup analysis to see if the causal effect of that intervention varies by the *observed* levels of some additional variable. For example, we could randomize home nursing visits versus standard of care to prevent secondary heart attacks after a first heart attack but then look to see if the causal effect of home nursing visits on the outcome was different in (for example) older compared with younger participants. In this latter case, we would not attempt to estimate a causal effect of age per se, but only examine whether the causal effects of the randomized intervention *varied* with age.

Why do we perform subgroup analysis? Discovering that an intervention works far better in one observed group than another (e.g., a smoking cessation intervention works far better in women than men) may help targeting of the intervention subsequently, as well as help to give us a sense of how generalizable our findings are to other populations. However, this latter point is complex, and subgroup analyses should not be assumed to be valid in specific external target populations without close attention and, indeed, additional assumptions.

Often randomized trials will publish their analytic protocols ahead of time, and critical subgroup analyses will be included in those protocols; however, typical clinical trials have low statistical power for most subgroup analyses (which, by their nature, split the main study data into distinct parts) unless they are powered specifically for those analyses.

5.5.2 Factorial Trials

In a subgroup analysis, there is one intervention, and then a secondary covariate: we examine the effect of the intervention within levels of the covariate but not effects of the covariate per se. Thus, there is a strong distinction between the intervention and the secondary covariate in the subgroup analysis. In contrast, in a factorial trial, there are two (or more, but usually only two) *co-equal interventions*: both are randomized, both can be interpreted as causal effects, and we can identify the joint causal effects of the two.

Specifically, factorial trials are those in which two entirely separate treatments are randomized, usually independently. For example, considering again a trial of interventions to prevent second heart attack among survivors of a first heart attack, we might randomize monthly home nursing visits versus standard of care but also randomize use of daily beta-blocker versus placebo. In such a case, we can imagine a 2 × 2 table of trial arms, shown in Table 5.8. In a factorial trial we

Table 5.8 POSSIBLE 1-YEAR RISK DIFFERENCES FROM A FACTORIAL OF BETA-BLOCKER VERSUS PLACEBO AND HOME NURSING VISITS VERSUS STANDARD OF CARE, COMPARING RISK OF SECONDARY HEART ATTACK

Risk of second MI		**Clinical**	
		Home nursing	Standard of care
Drug	Beta-blocker	0.08	0.15
	Placebo	0.18	0.20

can identify the effects of each intervention but also identify their joint effects: if the two interventions are synergistic (or antagonistic) in some way, we may see a larger (or smaller) effect of the two together than we would each separately.

Consider Table 5.8, where we show the risk of the outcome under each of four trial arms in a 2 × 2 factorial design. When both interventions are valued 0 (e.g., standard of care in both cases), the 1-year risk of the outcome is 20%. When someone receives clinical standard of care but also receives a beta-blocker, the 1-year risk of the outcome is 15% (risk difference −5%); when someone receives monthly home nursing visits and no beta-blocker, the 1 -year risk of the outcome is 18% (risk difference −2%); and when someone receives both interventions, the 1-year risk of the outcome is 8% (risk difference −12%). Thus, the risk with the two interventions combined is 12 absolute percentage points lower than in the absence of both interventions. Moreover we see clearly that the joint effect is substantially further from the null (or, greater in magnitude) than we would expect from each intervention separately (which might be −5% + −2% = −7% total impact rather than −12%). Such results might be expected in reality if, for example, the key role of the home nursing visits is to encourage long-term adherence to the beta-blocker—and so, in absence of the beta-blocker, the nursing visits make little difference, and, in absence of home nursing visits, adherence to the beta-blocker drops off substantially over time.

5.5.3 Causal Interaction (Joint Causal Effects) Versus Effect Measure Modification

The distinction between factorial trials, in which we investigate a joint causal effect, and subgroup analysis, in which we investigate whether a single causal effect differs between observed levels of an additional variable, is an important one and a distinction we will carry into observational data analysis as well. Specifically, this difference corresponds to the distinction drawn in observational data between causal interactions and effect measure modification (see Chapter 6).

5.6 SUMMARY

There are numerous strengths to randomized trials: they provide an excellent basis for estimation of causal effects within the trial population due to their unambiguous temporal sequence (exposure precedes outcome), their ability to ensure exchangeability (on measured and unmeasured confounders) in expectation via randomization, and the fact that they ensure both positivity and little to no treatment variation by design.

At the same time, however, causal effects estimated in trials may not generalize to target populations of interest, trials themselves are expensive and often difficult to organize, and trials remain vulnerable to loss to follow-up and other issues. Trials are often limited in being able to assess only shorter term outcomes and, of course, can only help us assess the causal effects of factors which can be ethically, and practically, randomized.

In Chapter 6, we shall see how prospective observational cohort studies can remedy at least some of these limitations of randomized trials while being themselves limited by several key factors.

5.7 REVIEWING A PUBLISHED REPORT OF A RANDOMIZED TRIAL

A comprehensive guide to reviewing reports of randomized trials is beyond the scope of this book, but we do wish to offer several thoughts to readers about important questions to ask when reading the results of a randomized trial.

We suggest that when reviewing a published report of a randomized trial, some critical questions to consider include (but are by no means limited to) the following.

1. What is the question the investigators are trying to answer? What are the implications of the answer to that question for decisions about treatment or policy?
2. What is the target population—the population in whom the results are meant to apply? Is the target population described explicitly or implied—if the latter, how? Do you think the baseline risk of the outcome is similar in the trial population and the target population? What subgroup effects were investigated in the report? Were they prespecified or ad hoc, and were substantial differences found by subgroups?
3. What is the treatment (intervention, exposure)? How was the treatment randomized? If there was no blinding, why not? Did the measured covariates show good balance across the arms of the trial (was randomization "successful"); and, if not, what are the implications (Senn, 2013)? Is the treatment being randomized something that can be scaled up into clinical or public health use quickly, and, if not, how can we relate the treatment tested in this report to a treatment that *could* be scaled up? Is this a treatment for which adherence is important to measure, and, if so, did they measure adherence? (And how good was adherence?)

4. What is the outcome (including in what timeframe), and how was it measured? Is there the possibility for mismeasurement or missing outcome data? If there was missing data, how did the authors deal with it?

5. Did the authors perform a compliance-corrected analysis in addition to an ITT analysis? Do the two analyses convey different overall messages or implications?

6. What is the estimated effect, and what are the implications of that estimated effect in the context of previous work on the subject? Did the trial confirm or contradict previous work, and why might that be?

REFERENCES

Allison, P. D. (2010). *Survival analysis using SAS: A practical guide* (2nd ed.). Cary, NC: SAS Press.

Amrhein, V., Greenland, S., & McShane, B. (2019). Scientists rise up against statistical significance. *Nature, 567*(7748), 305–307. doi:10.1038/d41586-019-00857-9

Bland, J. M., & Altman, D. G. (1998). Survival probabilities (the Kaplan-Meier method). *BMJ, 317*(7172), 1572.

Ford, I., & Norrie, J. (2016). Pragmatic trials. *New England Journal of Medicine, 375*(5), 454–463. doi:10.1056/NEJMra1510059

Hernán, M. A., & Hernández-Díaz, S. (2012). Beyond the intention-to-treat in comparative effectiveness research. *Clinical Trials, 9*(1), 48–55.

Hernán, M. A., Alonso, A., Logan, R., Grodstein, F., Michels, K. B., Willett, W. C., . . . Robins, J. M. (2008). Observational studies analyzed like randomized experiments: An application to postmenopausal hormone therapy and coronary heart disease. *Epidemiology, 19*(6), 766–779. doi:10.1097/EDE.0b013e3181875e61

Hofmeyr, G. J., Morrison, C. S., Baeten, J. M., Chipato, T., Donnell, D., Gichangi, P., . . . Team, E. T. (2017). Rationale and design of a multi-center, open-label, randomised clinical trial comparing HIV incidence and contraceptive benefits in women using three commonly-used contraceptive methods (the ECHO study). *Gates Open Research, 1*, 17. doi:10.12688/gatesopenres.12775.1

Kaplan, E. L., & Meier, P. (1958). Nonparametric estimation from incomplete observations. *Journal of the American Statistical Association, 53*(282), 457–481.

Lee, P. Y., Alexander, K. P., Hammill, B. G., Pasquali, S. K., & Peterson, E. D. (2001). Representation of elderly persons and women in published randomized trials of acute coronary syndromes. *Journal of the American Medical Association, 286*(6), 708–713.

Little, R. J. A., & Rubin, D. B. (2002). *Statistical analysis with missing data* (2nd ed.). New York: John Wiley.

Polis, C. B., Curtis, K. M., Hannaford, P. C., Phillips, S. J., Chipato, T., Kiarie, J. N., . . . Steyn, P. S. (2016). An updated systematic review of epidemiological evidence on hormonal contraceptive methods and HIV acquisition in women. *AIDS, 30*(17), 2665–2683. doi:10.1097/QAD.0000000000001228

Polis, C. B., Westreich, D., Balkus, J. E., Heffron, R., & Participants of the HCHIVOAM. (2013). Assessing the effect of hormonal contraception on HIV acquisition in observational data: Challenges and recommended analytic approaches. *AIDS*, *27*(Suppl 1), S35–S43. doi:10.1097/QAD.0000000000000036

Poole, C. (2001). Low P-values or narrow confidence intervals: Which are more durable? *Epidemiology*, *12*(3), 291–294.

Powney, M., Williamson, P., Kirkham, J., & Kolamunnage-Dona, R. (2014). A review of the handling of missing longitudinal outcome data in clinical trials. *Trials*, *15*, 237. doi:10.1186/1745-6215-15-237

Senn, S. (2013). Seven myths of randomisation in clinical trials. *Statistical Medicine*, *32*(9), 1439–1450. doi:10.1002/sim.5713

Shadish, W., Cook, T., & Campbell, D. (2002). *Experimental and quasi-experimental designs for generalized causal inference.* New York: Houghton Mifflin.

Stang, A., Poole, C., & Kuss, O. (2010). The ongoing tyranny of statistical significance testing in biomedical research. *European Journal of Epidemiology*, *25*(4), 225–230. doi:10.1007/s10654-010-9440-x

Westreich, D., Edwards, J. K., Lesko, C. R., Cole, S. R., & Stuart, E. A. (2019). Target validity and the hierarchy of study designs. *American Journal of Epidemiology*, *188*(2), 438–443. doi:10.1093/aje/kwy228

6

Observational Cohort Studies

In contrast to a randomized trial, an observational cohort study is one in which the investigator *observes* a *group of participants* with varying levels of *an exposure* (such as a pharmaceutical product, environmental condition, or health behavior) and then follows up those participants for a period of time to examine the incidence of *one or more specified outcomes*.

Observational studies are widely considered inferior to randomized trials for establishing causality, an idea encoded in numerous hierarchies of evidence or study designs. This (in our opinion) is largely because *well-designed and well-executed* trials generally have strong internal validity, whereas observational studies may be subject to challenges to their internal validity, especially confounding, and for other reasons as well. However, observational studies often can make a stronger claim to external validity because they are often more representative of target populations of interest (see also Chapter 9). Thus an observational study that uses reasonable methods to address internal validity threats may provide more valid estimates of what would happen as a result of taking action in a specific target population than would a randomized trial (Westreich, Edwards, Lesko, Cole, & Stuart, 2019).

At the beginning of the previous chapter, we described a randomized trial to understand whether a fictional vaccine prevents heart attack. We explained how we might flip a coin to assign some participants to receive the vaccine and others to receive a placebo and then follow-up participants to see who experienced the outcome. Consider instead that we *observed* whether participants chose, on their own, to take the vaccine or not (with no one receiving placebo), and then studied how incidence of heart attack differed between those who took the vaccine and those who did not.

Such a study would typically be called a *prospective observational cohort study*, and one key concern in such a study would be that the incidence of heart attack could differ between those receiving the vaccine and those not receiving of the vaccine, not due to the effect of the vaccine itself but at least in part because those who choose the vaccine are likely systematically different from those who choose not to receive the vaccine.

Epidemiology by Design: A Causal Approach to the Health Sciences. Daniel Westreich, Oxford University Press (2020). © Oxford University Press.
DOI: 10.1093/oso/9780190665760.001.0001

6.1 MECHANICS

As with a randomized trial, a deep dive into the mechanics of how to organize and run an observational cohort study is beyond our scope. Here, we dwell on (i) methodologically important decisions in initiating and running a cohort study and also (ii) key differences from randomized trials. We leave out discussion of creation of study protocols, obtaining institutional review board (IRB) approval, and so on.

6.1.1 Finding a Study Question (an Exposure/Outcome Combination)

When is a question better suited to an observational cohort study than a randomized trial? First and foremost, when randomizing the exposure of interest is practically difficult or ethically unthinkable. For example, pregnancy can impact risk of depression, but the notion of randomizing pregnancy is absurdly unethical on its face (in addition to being practically impossible). If one wants to study the impact of pregnancy on depression, one could (however) observe individuals who become pregnant and follow-up those individuals for depression-related outcomes, comparing them to women who do not become pregnant. Likewise, smoking, asbestos exposure, recreational drug use, trauma—these are all exposures which are unethical to randomize, and so observational approaches are necessary.

Another factor that might make a question more amenable to observational, rather than randomized, approaches is if we believe that the fact of someone choosing an intervention for themselves may be important to the effect that intervention has. For example, most people, given a choice between a low-fat diet (give up cheese) and a low-carb diet (give up soda) have strong feelings about which they would prefer. While we might want to look at the effect of random assignment to one diet or the other on weight loss, we might also be interested in seeing the effects of each diet compared to the other when each is chosen by the individual. The latter case—which is possible in an observational setting—might be desirable if people are more likely to stick to a diet they choose rather than one to which they are assigned.

6.1.2 Selecting a Target Population and Study Sample

As with randomized trials, it is ideal to identify up front the target population about which you want to learn with the study and then select a study sample that will be informative about that target population. On the latter point, while informed consent must be obtained to enroll participants into a cohort (with some exceptions, such as cases of routinely collected de-identified data), some individuals may be more likely to participate in a cohort study than a randomized trial. The bar for participation may be lower because in an observational setting no random experiment will be conducted on participants—leaving choices about treatment in the hands of participants. This in turn may mean that the typical cohort study will more closely represent potential target populations than the typical randomized trial (see also discussion in Chapter 9).

6.1.3 Assessing Exposure, Covariate, and Outcome Status

As in a randomized trial, clear and usable definitions of exposure and outcome are desirable in a cohort study and, when possible, should be assessed in a blinded way or by neutral evaluators (who are not invested in study results). Poor or unclear definition of the exposure, in particular, has implications for the consistency assumption (see later discussion) and thus may impact the ability to make causal inference with findings from a study.

While randomized trials collect covariate information (and show that information in "Table 1"), randomization ensures that intention-to-treat (ITT) analysis will generally be valid without any effort to account for covariates, in a "crude" or unadjusted analysis. In an observational setting, lack of randomization means that such crude analyses are likely to be biased due to confounding: thus, in observational settings we must collect confounders in order to control for confounding. Thus, we start our covariate collection process by developing a causal directed acyclic graph (DAG) for our exposure–outcome relationship based on previously published literature. Under the assumption of a correctly specified DAG containing exposure, outcome, and confounders of the exposure–outcome relationship, as well as other covariates of interest, the DAG can be analyzed to obtain a list of covariates that will be sufficient to control confounding in analysis.

6.2 CAUSAL INFERENCE IN OBSERVATIONAL COHORT STUDIES

As noted earlier, there is a broad consensus within epidemiology and biostatistics that observational studies are inferior for obtaining estimates of causal effects compared to randomized trials. This consensus is largely due to a focus on confounding, although challenges to treatment variation irrelevance in observational settings are underappreciated in this argument. This consensus view has serious limitations, but we defer these discussions for the moment. Here, we discuss causal identification conditions within the context of observational cohort studies.

6.2.1 Causal Identification Conditions

Here we address temporality, conditional exchangeability with positivity, consistency, and measurement error.

6.2.1.1 TEMPORALITY

For an exposure to have caused an outcome, it must have occurred prior to the outcome. Cohort studies ensure temporality by enrolling only participants who have not developed the outcome at enrollment. However, ensuring temporality by design can be tricky because the key causal exposure may not always have occurred at the time we recorded it, thus leading to issues with *latency*. For example, suppose we wish to use cancer mortality as a measure of cancer incidence because the former is easy to measure: in such a case, we should not consider exposures measured after cancer incidence but before cancer mortality as potential causes of the cancer—such exposures would violate temporality. Somewhat related, see discussions of lead-time bias and length-time bias in Chapter 4, as well as Box 6.1 on left-truncation bias, which is also related in part to timing of events.

Regarding issues of time, there are two main types of observational cohort studies discussed in the literature: prospective and retrospective cohorts. While the terminology is frequently confusing, the distinction is usually drawn on when the data were collected. In a *prospective cohort*, we enroll individuals, collect information at enrollment, and then follow them forward in time to collect outcome data. In a *retrospective cohort*, we identify a group of individuals who did not have the outcome of interest at some point in the past, and we collect information about their history through interviews or existing data records.

It is important, in this discussion, to note that the timing of the *measurement* of a condition or variable does not establish the timing of the *occurrence* of that condition or variable. For example, genotypes can be measured at any age, with

---

Box 6.1

LEFT TRUNCATION BIAS

It is sometimes the case in an observational study that we use *prevalent* conditions as our exposure: for example, at the time of initiation of antiretroviral therapy, we compare individuals with prevalent tuberculosis (TB) to those without prevalent TB and follow-up all individuals for an outcome of mortality. While on its face this situation is one in which exposure (TB) precedes the outcome (mortality), a bias can arise because some people with TB and HIV will die of TB before managing to initiate antiretroviral therapy and thus are never considered in analysis. If you want to know the causal effect of getting TB on survival post therapy initiation, those people who died of TB—but you never observed—are a vital part of the causal story.

This is known as *left truncation bias*: "left" in that it occurred earlier on the left-to-right timeline and "truncation" in that we do not observe events or indeed entire individuals due to their timing. Left truncation bias can be seen as a problem with temporality and exchangeability, and, as an exchangeability problem, it can be thought of as both confounding (in that, since we do not see the beginning of exposure, we cannot control confounding at the moment of first exposure) and selection bias (because we do not observe all individuals in whom we want to make inference).

confidence about when they were fixed. On the other hand, cognition measured at age 75 may reflect changes that took place 10 or 15 years earlier; the same might be true for exposures and outcomes highly correlated across periods of an individual's life, such as poverty or body mass index. As well, collecting information retrospectively may lead to issues with reliability of self-report (which may deteriorate over time) but not with administrative records, which should not deteriorate.

6.2.1.2 EXCHANGEABILITY

As noted repeatedly, the lack of exchangeability (specifically in the form of confounding) is the best-known and best-understood difference between causality in randomized trials and in observational studies, and observational studies cannot typically guarantee exchangeability between exposure groups. This is perhaps best expressed with a causal diagram: we show examples of DAGs for observational studies later. In general, the lack of exchangeability in observational studies is referred to as *confounding bias* and *selection bias* and is broadly what people mean when they say "correlation is not causation." Although we hasten to remind you that correlation is not *unrelated* to causation, either.

Observational studies thus rarely if ever display *unconditional* exchangeability (Chapters 3 and 5). To estimate causal effects in observational studies, it is usually necessary to make an assumption of *conditional exchangeability* and control for confounding by conditioning on variables identified from a DAG. Conditioning, here, is usually in observational settings achieved by including those variables in a regression model, a form of "adjusting" for those variables (see Sections 6.3 and 6.6); other methods include stratifying, restricting, and standardizing. As soon as we are conditioning on any variables, however, we must grapple with potential issues in *positivity*.

6.2.1.3 POSITIVITY AND EXPOSURE OPPORTUNITY

Since causal effect estimation in observational studies generally requires conditional exchangeability, it likewise requires us to consider positivity. Again, positivity is that the probability of exposure and nonexposure (or any level of the exposure, if there are more than two levels) is greater than zero for every level of every variable being modeled or otherwise accounted for. As noted in Chapter 3, we sometimes refer to the combination of exchangeability given measured covariates along with positivity as a single assumption: *conditional exchangeability with positivity*.

Closely related to positivity is the issue of exposure opportunity: we should only study people who can, at least in theory, experience all the exposure conditions under study. But in an observational context, we sometimes include individuals with no exposure opportunity. For example, in a study of the impact of pregnancy on some outcome, we might by accident include women who are infertile and thus could never experience pregnancy: these women would have no exposure opportunity. A causal effect estimate which includes those women is ill-defined and difficult to interpret.

6.2.1.4 CONSISTENCY

Recall that in a randomized trial, treatment is typically assigned in the same way (by protocol) for all participants, and thus treatment *assignment* varies only minimally, although there may be substantial variation in how treatment is actually received. This second issue is generally true of observational studies, in which exposure or treatment is rarely under the control of the investigator. The way people are exposed in an observational study may vary enormously, and this variation may prove a significant barrier to causal inference based on the analysis of observational data—especially if we have failed to measure the exposure route! For example, if the exposure is aspirin use, then, even among individuals who take aspirin every day, dose of aspirin (1 baby aspirin, or 2?) may vary—and such variation may be important to the effect of the aspirin. With sufficiently good recording of dose, investigators may deal with such variation in analysis; thus, dose–response relationships, when ignored, provide an important subcategory of consistency concerns in observational studies. In addition, this formulation suggests a possibly useful connection between consistency (or treatment variation) and measurement error.

A related problem is that there are numerous exposures whose causal effects are of interest and which seem conceptually clear but which cannot be randomized even in principle and which are quite difficult to precisely define. For example, factors including race, sex, and socioeconomic status all pose substantial problems for the consistency assumption (Rehkopf, Glymour, & Osypuk, 2016; VanderWeele & Robinson, 2014).

6.2.1.5 MEASUREMENT ERROR

As in randomized studies, measurement error is possible and indeed likely, and, if present, it will impair our ability to estimate causal effects accurately. By convention and design, measurement error of exposure and outcome are often more present and salient in observational studies compared to randomized trials. By convention, we mean that while there is no barrier to assessing outcomes as accurately in an observational setting as in a randomized trial, randomized trials often do a better job at this task. By design, we mean that treatment assignment can be measured without error in a way that actual treatment cannot.

In addition, observational studies near-invariably require additional variables to be collected so that conditional exchangeability can be achieved: these variables must also be correctly measured.

6.2.2 Causal Directed Acyclic Graphs

In an observational study, people are exposed for a variety of reasons, some of which may be related to the outcome under study. For example, consider a study in which we are trying to determine whether (short-term or recent) smoking causes car accidents. If we randomized smoking status, then with perfect compliance (such that only those assigned to smoke actually smoke), in expectation smokers and

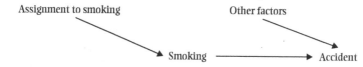

Figure 6.1 Directed acyclic graph for a randomized trial of smoking.

nonsmokers will have similar distributions of measured and unmeasured covariates and therefore similar pre-smoking risks of the outcome. Thus, in Figure 6.1, we see that Assignment to smoking is the only thing that affects true smoking.

In a nonrandomized setting, it is often the case that drinking alcohol leads to more smoking. Since drinking alcohol may raise the risk of car accidents (Figure 6.2), smokers may have a higher baseline risk of car accidents than nonsmokers independent of smoking itself due to the effect of alcohol. As such, unconditional exchangeability generally cannot be assumed in observational settings except under specific conditions (see Quasi-Experiments in Chapter 8). Instead, in an observational study, we try to obtain conditional exchangeability by controlling for confounding, as we describe later.

In Chapter 3, we described how to identify open backdoor paths and a sufficient set of covariates to account for confounding. In Figure 6.1, there are no such paths because there are no arrows into Smoking except for the random assignment. In Figure 6.2, there is an open backdoor path from Smoking ← Drinking alcohol → Accident risk, and thus we must account for Drinking in any analysis to ensure we are free of confounding.

Using a DAG to identify confounders, and then accounting for those confounders in analysis, can help to clarify thinking about how to achieve exchangeability between exposure groups. We say "help" rather than "guarantee" because we can only achieve exchangeability insofar as we can identify, correctly measure, and correctly model the effect of all confounders. Since there might always be unmeasured (or poorly measured) confounders or errors in the models or methods we use to identify or correct them, we can *never* guarantee exchangeability by analytic means.

6.3 ADDRESSING CONFOUNDING IN OBSERVATIONAL COHORT STUDIES

The steps in cohort analysis very much echo those in a randomized trial analysis: the data should be frozen for analysis, coded, and analyzed. At the time of

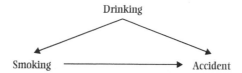

Figure 6.2 Directed acyclic graph for an observational study of smoking.

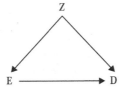

Figure 6.3 Directed acyclic graph illustrating the classic confounding triangle.

this publication, there is ongoing debate around whether all observational cohort analyses should be preregistered prior to the conduct of a study. While preregistration can help to improve transparency of analysis even when it is not strictly adhered to, it is perhaps more important to understand how to report and interpret our uncertainty correctly; preregistration can help with this, but does not guarantee it.

6.3.1 Control of Confounding

A central step in analysis of cohort data is dealing with confounding. As noted earlier, the first step in this process is representing your existing knowledge and assumptions, for example, by drawing a DAG—ideally, before data collection begin—so that it is clear ahead of time which confounders are important before it is too late to get information on them. Here, we assume that we are at the analysis stage of a study, confounders have been identified, and information on them collected. Now: What does confounding look like, and how do we account for it?

Consider the DAG (Figure 6.3) in which the effect of E on D is confounded by Z (because there is an open backdoor path, $E \leftarrow Z \rightarrow D$). Sample data consistent with this DAG are shown in Table 6.1, in three 2×2 tables: one in which we see the

Table 6.1 DATA CONSISTENT WITH THE DIRECTED ACYCLIC
GRAPH (DAG) IN FIGURE 6.3

All Z	D yes	D no	Total	Risk
Exposed	700	1,300	2,000	0.350
Unexposed	300	1,700	2,000	0.150
Total	1,000	3,000	4,000	0.250
$Z = 1$ only	D yes	D no	Total	Risk
Exposed	100	400	500	0.200
Unexposed	150	1,350	1,500	0.100
Total	250	1,750	2,000	0.125
$Z = 0$ only	D yes	D no	Total	Risk
Exposed	600	900	1,500	0.400
Unexposed	150	350	500	0.300
Total	750	1,250	2,000	0.375

effect of E on D while ignoring the confounder Z (labeled "All Z"), one table for the effect of E on D when $Z = 1$, and one table for the effect of E on D when $Z = 0$. For the purposes of this example, we ignore any statistical uncertainty.

We note several links between the DAG and the 2 × 2 tables. The DAG implies that there is an effect of Z on E, which should be reflected in a different distribution of E by levels of Z in the 2 × 2 tables: and, indeed, where $Z = 1$, 500/2,000 (25%) of participants are exposed, and where $Z = 0$, 1,500/2,000 (75%) of participants are exposed. Likewise, the DAG implies a direct effect of Z on D, which is consistent with the data in the 2 × 2 tables: among the exposed ($E = 1$ only), the risk of the outcome in $Z = 1$ is 0.2 and the risk of the outcome in $Z = 0$ is 0.4, for a risk difference (RD) of −0.2.

A final connection to draw between the data in Table 6.1 and DAGs is illustrated by Figure 6.4: the data in Table 6.1 are fully consistent not just with the DAG in Figure 6.3, but *also* with Figure 6.4 in which Z *is not a confounder but a mediator of the* $E{\to}D$ *relationship*. This is a subtle point: these 2 × 2 tables are fully consistent with a situation in which Z is a mediator. In such a scenario, to estimate the total effect of E on D, we would *not* control for Z. Thus, if you are presented with 2 × 2 tables that look like those in Table 6.1, you cannot tell *from the* 2 × 2 *tables alone* whether to account for Z or to ignore it and look in the combined, or crude, data. You need some prior knowledge of the time-ordering of E and Z—such as the knowledge encoded in a DAG—to determine what role Z plays. If Z truly is a mediator, and you want the total effect of E on D, the best way to proceed is to simply collapse over levels of Z and take the crude RD: in Table 6.1, this would mean calculating the RD from the top 2 × 2 table ("All Z"), as 0.35 − 0.15 = 0.20. (Yes: this will be on the test.)

In the case where we really do have a confounder or confounders, however (e.g., if Figure 6.3 is true), we must deal analytically with the variable(s) in question. Several quantitative methods are possible here, which we might broadly break into two categories: first, stratification, and second, stratification followed by recombination of strata. In the second category we can take numerous approaches, including Mantel-Haenszel methods (see later discussion), regression, and standardization. In the following section, we briefly describe each of these approaches conceptually; in later sections, we explore some analytic approaches in more detail. We then briefly describe a third, more design-based method for dealing with confounding: matching.

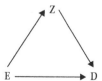

Figure 6.4 Directed acyclic graph illustrating the classic mediation triangle.

6.3.2 Stratification Approaches

Suppose we have an exposure (*E*) and an outcome (*D*) and a confounder (*Z*); suppose further that *Z* has two levels, 0 (absent) and 1 (present). *Stratification*, broadly, occurs is when we estimate the effect of *E* on *D* among those with $Z = 0$ and separately estimate the effect of *E* on *D* among those with $Z = 1$. A close variant of this approach is *restriction*, in which we restrict our analysis to only one level of a confounder instead of both (or all) simultaneously. For a group of individuals all with the same level of *Z* (e.g., the 1,000 people with $Z = 1$), there is no causal effect of level of *Z* on exposure or disease outcome and so no confounding by *Z*. Interpretation of such a calculation is obviously limited in that our estimated causal effect can only apply to those with $Z = 1$.

6.3.3 Recombination of Strata

While making stratum-specific estimates is straightforward, we may wish to produce a single estimate of effect over all *Z*. In such a case we will need to recombine the two strata using a weighted average. Which weights are used to recombine strata-specific estimates varies from method to method and the weights used help define the underlying quantity being estimated. Here, we briefly describe several approaches to recombining strata

6.3.3.1 MANTEL-HAENSZEL METHODS

There are numerous ways to approach the recombining of strata: the first taught in many epidemiology courses is the *Mantel-Haenszel* (sometimes *Cochran-Mantel-Haenszel*) approach. In essence the Mantel-Haenszel method does exactly what we just outlined: takes the effect in each level of *Z* and then combines across levels of *Z* using calculated weights. Returning to the example data shown in Table 6.1, it is easy to see that the RD in both the $Z = 0$ and $Z = 1$ groups is 0.10, and so combining the two strata is trivial (any weighted average of 0.10 and 0.10 is equal to 0.10); this approach works similarly in more than two categories, though not with continuous variables. A general point here is that the Mantel-Haenszel is recommended when the effect in each stratum is essentially the same: if not exactly the same (as in our example), then similar enough that a single summary of the two does not erase critical information. (What is "critical" is a subject matter–specific decision.) Some details of the Mantel-Haenszel approach are given in section 6.6.1.

6.3.3.2 REGRESSION

Another well-known stratification approach to dealing with confounding is *regression*. Regression rests on same key assumption as the Mantel-Haenszel approach: specifically, that of constant effects of exposure on outcome within strata of the covariates. Regression models typically also rely on numerous other assumptions. There are entire textbooks dedicated to understanding regression analysis in both statistical and intuitive terms; here, we note only that, conceptually, drawing a regression line is intuitively very much like the "$y = mx + b$" exercises many readers will have explored in seventh-grade math class. In addition, regression analysis can help deal with continuous variables in ways that Mantel-Haenszel methods cannot. See Box 6.2 for an important caution regarding the interpretation of results from a regression analysis.

6.3.4 Standardization

Standardization uses different weights than either Mantel-Haenszel or regression approaches. While the weights used in the two previously described methods change with the statistical information (e.g., the precision) of each stratum-specific estimate, standardization uses weights derived from simple proportions of the population, often by category of the confounders. Application of these weights allows us to estimate population average effects, which often have a useful public health interpretation.

For example, an age-standardized mortality rate—which many readers may have heard of—is simply a way of identifying an expected population average mortality rate absent the influence of age. Specifically, suppose we want to compare the 1-year risk of death for residents of Maine to that of Utah.[1] As it turns out, the median age of Maine is (at this writing) substantially higher than that of Utah—so the risk of death in a given year might be higher in Maine than in Utah because of the age distribution, rather than because of any other differences between the states.

To compare more honestly—absent the influence of age—we might ask different questions: For example, had Utah—counter to fact—had the same age distribution as Maine, what difference would we expect to observe between 1-year of death in counterfactual Utah and in Maine? In such a situation, there would no longer be any association between age and state, and so any differences between the two states can be attributed to something other than age. We have just described what is commonly called *direct standardization*; in contrast, *indirect standardization* occurs when instead we take the age-specific mortality rates from Maine and apply them to the population distribution of Utah.

All these methods are simply an application of weighted averaging. Likewise, a related approach to standardization is *inverse probability weighting* (IPW). IPW is often thought of as an "advanced" method in epidemiology, but in fact is relatively straightforward to implement and is closely related to methods for survey sampling and reweighting as well as standardization. Properly applying IPW to a population, as with all forms of standardization, creates a "pseudo-population" in which exposure is not associated with confounders, assuming those confounders are properly measured and modeled. (In our age-standardized mortality example, "state and its healthcare" could be thought of as the exposure and "age" was the confounder.)

---

1. We have no agenda here regarding the relative healthcare systems of the two states.

Box 6.2

The Table 2 Fallacy

Typical regression analysis does not distinguish between the exposure variable and confounding variables in the statistical model and thus can produce estimates of the RD (or RR, odds ratio, etc.) for all variables in the regression model. In the preceding model, we calculated β_0, β_1, and β_2. As well, there is a tendency in the epidemiologic and biomedical literature to report all beta coefficients from a regression model except the intercept—so in the preceding model, β_1 and β_2 — in a single table. This implicitly, and sometimes explicitly, suggests that all these coefficients can be interpreted as causal effects of the exposure on the outcome. They should not be: such an interpretation is the Table 2 Fallacy (Westreich & Greenland, 2013). There are two problems with this (quite typical approach). First, examining Figure 6.6a, notice that the effect of Z on D has two parts: first, the direct effect shown in the arrow from Z directly to D, and second, the indirect effect of Z on D which goes through E. In the analysis of data corresponding to Figure 6.6a, then, β_1 will represent the total effect of E on D, but β_2 will represent effect of Z on D which is not mediated by E (i.e., "the direct effect of Z on D not mediated by E"). If we wanted the *total effect* of Z on D, our regression model would not include E at all: for example, for Figure 6.6a, our model might be $\Pr(D) = \beta_0 + \beta_2 Z$, which omits the E term. As it is, both β_2 and β_1 are causal effects, but they are of different types (direct, indirect): putting the two effects side by side in a single table implies to the reader that they are to be interpreted similarly.

Worse, however, compare Figure 6.6a to 6.6b, where our goal is to estimate the effect of E on D. For either diagram, all open backdoor paths between E and D are closed by controlling for Z; thus, for either diagram, the original regression model ($E(D) = \Pr(D) = \beta_0 + \beta_1 E + \beta_2 Z$) is sufficient to deal with confounding of the $E \rightarrow D$ relationship and there is no need to condition on U. However, in Figure 6.6b, the $Z \rightarrow D$ relationship is seen to be confounded by U, in that there is an open backdoor path from Z to D through U. If Figure 6.6b is the truth, but we fit the original regression model not including U, then our report of the $Z \rightarrow D$ beta coefficient as an effect estimate not only misleads the reader as described earlier, but furthermore also may be a biased estimate of that direct effect because of uncontrolled confounding of the $Z \rightarrow D$ relationship by U.

Reporting beta coefficients for covariates/confounders in the same table and format as a main effect estimate has the potential to confuse readers into thinking these coefficients are estimates of causal effect. How—and whether—to report such beta coefficients should be considered carefully.

In a DAG, this is the equivalent of removing the arrow from the confounder to the exposure (in Figure 6.3, removing the $Z{\rightarrow}E$ arrow). Recall that randomization of E would also remove the $Z{\rightarrow}E$ arrow. Specifically, under randomization, we would introduce a new node and arrow (as in the "Assignment to smoking" node in Figure 6.1); only with perfect compliance with treatment assignment would the estimated effect of treatment *assignment* be equal to the estimated effect of treatment per se. Similarly, only under perfect compliance could we ignore the randomization node and arrow into E. Of course, while randomization removes all arrows into the exposure (except for the randomization arrow itself), IPW approaches can only remove arrows into the exposure from known and measured covariates—and even then, only under correct specification of any necessary models.

6.3.4.1 COMPARISON OF METHODS

All three approaches just described assume that we want to take a weighted average over the levels of Z. As noted earlier, the weights used in Mantel-Haenszel and regression approaches make sense chiefly if the effect of E on D is "the same" in each level of Z; that is, if the effects in each level of Z are similar enough (*homogeneous*) that no potentially important information is lost in combining them. If the effect of E on D is sufficiently different (*heterogeneous*) across levels of Z that those differences have public health or clinical implications, then, in general, people reading your manuscript may wish you to report that fact, rather than simply averaging over levels of Z and ignoring the heterogeneity. Alternatively, they may wish to use a statistical test to examine the assumption of homogeneity. In contrast, standardization is a way of side-stepping questions of heterogeneity of effects to get a simple average effect of E on D in the observed sample—given the observed distribution of Z—without assuming homogeneity of effects.

6.3.5 Matching

Confounding can also be controlled through matching. The idea of matching is to create pairs (or groups) of individuals who are similar in key ways but differ in exposure conditions: for example, for every exposed 25-year-old, find an unexposed 25-year-old. Within strata of matched pairs (or larger groups of matched individuals), individuals are generally considered as good as randomized with respect to the matching variables (only; not randomized with respect to all covariates), and therefore, within each stratum we can assume no confounding by the matching variables. Analysis of matched data can be complex, however, and we do not dwell on analytic approaches here. We do note in passing that propensity scores, which are closely related to the IPW approach, are a popular way of matching on multiple variables at once (Joffe & Rosenbaum, 1999; Rosenbaum & Rubin, 1983).

6.4 INTERACTION AND EFFECT
MEASURE MODIFICATION

Recall from our discussion of trials the difference between a factorial trial and a subgroup analysis: in a factorial trial, we randomize two distinct interventions and examine the joint causal effects of the two interventions. In a subgroup analysis, we examine whether the causal effect of a single intervention varies between observed levels of an additional variable, where the additional variable is not randomized.

The same distinction exists, with some caveats, in observational settings. In observational data, we can simulate a factorial trial by assessing the causal effects of two independent and co-equal exposure (or treatment) conditions and then examining their joint causal effects. Estimates of the joint causal effects are often termed *interaction* (VanderWeele, 2009) though here we prefer the term *causal interaction* to distinguish from certain statistical phenomena (see later discussion). Such an observational analysis of joint causal effects must confront causal identification conditions for *both* exposures. That is, *both* exposure–outcome relationships must meet conditions of temporality, conditional exchangeability with positivity, consistency, and no measurement error (or an alternative set of assumptions) in order for the interaction analysis to yield results interpretable in terms of the joint causal effects of the two exposures.

We can likewise perform pseudo-subgroup analysis in observational data by asking whether a specific exposure has a different causal effect in the different observed levels of some additional variable. In such an observational analysis we generally say that we are looking for *effect measure modification*; like subgroup effects, effect measure modification is concerned with only a single potential causal effect. And just as subgroup analysis is unconcerned that the subgroup variable is not randomized, assessment of effect measure modification is not concerned with the causal identification assumptions for the modifying variable. As an example of effect measure modification, consider again the data shown in Table 6.1: when $Z = 1$, the risks are 0.20 and 0.10, for a risk ratio (RR) of 2.0; when $Z = 0$, the risks are 0.40 and 0.30, for a RR of 1.33. Note that we make no specific claims about the causal effects of Z on the outcome; here, we merely observe that the effect of exposure on disease is qualitatively different comparing the two levels of Z.

We delineate both causal interaction and effect measure modification from *statistical interaction*. Statistical interaction is a term relevant to regression modeling, when we create a variable by (in the simplest case) multiplying two other variables together: for example, we might have a variable for weight, a variable for age, and a variable for *weight times age*. The inclusion of this statistical interaction term allows the estimated effect of weight to differ with age (and vice versa). It is critical to understand that the results of a statistical analysis including a statistical interaction term may be interpreted as *either causal interaction or effect measure modification*, depending on what assumptions are made and particularly how confounding is dealt with in that analysis. And, of course, it might be

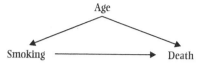

Figure 6.5 A simple directed acyclic graph for the effect of smoking on death, confounded by age.

that causal identification assumptions are not met for *any* variable in a particular regression model.

6.4.1 Confounding and Effect Measure Modification

In Figure 6.5, examining the impact of current smoking (any number of cigarettes) compared to current nonsmoking on death, we might be concerned about confounding by age: smoking prevalence changes with age, and age is a strong cause of death through various pathways. Consistent with this argument, in Figure 6.5, we would determine that age might confound the smoking–death relationship and adjust by age. However, we *also* might consider whether age is an *effect measure modifier* (EMM): if the impact of smoking on death is stronger among older people than among younger people, we might see substantial heterogeneity for the effect of smoking on death over a range of ages. How should we proceed?

This is a topic of debate among epidemiologists, some of which is beyond the scope of this book. One easy way forward is to consider whether—if there *were* effect measure modification—it would be of interest to the audience for your work. In this case, knowing if the RD for smoking is higher in older people than younger ones (for example), or in men than women, might be of interest. It could, for example, lead to an increase in resources devoted to smoking cessation among one group, rather than another, and more efficient use of resources. On the other hand, if the intervention for smoking is mass education through billboards, then knowing whether the RD is higher in (say) men compared with women is unlikely to help with public health policy making.

Thus, one possible way to proceed is as follows for each covariate Z (which is again assumed to have two levels, 0 and 1):

1. Would it be important to report EMM by Z, if it existed? If so, go to 2; else go to 3.
2. Look for EMM by Z.
    a. If EMM is present, report results separately by level of Z. (If Z is continuous, we could report at several values of Z; e.g., at quartiles of the values of Z.)
    b. If EMM is absent, go to 3.
3. Treat Z as a confounder and proceed.

Point 2a in the algorithm needs expansion: whether effect measure modification is present can be considered both a substantive question and a statistical one. If there is a meaningful difference between the values of the effect in $Z = 0$ and $Z = 1$, but that difference is statistically nonsignificant, it may or may not make sense to conclude that EMM is worth reporting.[2] Likewise if there is a very small and clinically meaningless difference between values, but that difference is statistically significant (e.g., as might be the case with vast amounts of data), it may not be worth reporting. In addition, it is important to realize that Z may still be a confounder, but we have side-stepped this concern by reporting only stratum-specific estimates of Z (i.e., by restriction).

On Point 3, it might be the case that Z is indeed an EMM, but it is not important. Here, we can proceed to analyze Z as a confounder. But in this case standardization approaches (e.g., IPWs) are likely preferable to stratification approaches such as Mantel-Haenszel methods because these latter methods typically assume that the effect of the exposure on the outcome is the same in each level of Z. Finally, we may wish to present both stratified and nonstratified results in a manuscript: Z may be an important EMM, but we might also like to use standardization to get a population average estimate.

The approach described in the preceding algorithm is by no means complete, but it is a good starting point for new epidemiologists; one other point to consider is the generalizability of the cohort study (see later discussion). One other, somewhat subtle point relevant to this discussion is expounded on in Section 6.4.3, "Most Confounders Are Modifiers."

6.4.2 Effect Measure Modification and Changing Baseline Risks

Consider a study of 10-year risk of death among individuals exposed to a particular industrial accident (say, a one-time chemical spill). Presume that the chemical spill was experienced by individuals essentially at random, so that we do not need to consider confounding at the moment. We study Population 1 as given in Table 6.2, in which the risk of heart attack among those unexposed to the chemical spill was 0.125; the risk among the exposed was 0.250. The 10-year RD is therefore 0.125, and the 10-year RR is 2.0.

We now consider Population 2, in which the baseline risk of heart attack (i.e., the risk among the unexposed) is substantially higher. This might be the case if there were more smokers in Population 2; note that in this scenario, smoking is not a confounder of the exposure–outcome relationship as seen by the equal chances of exposure (0.5) in both populations.

Now: What is the risk among the exposed in Population 2? We suspect that it will be higher than in Population 1 for the same sorts of reasons as the unexposed group in Population 2 has a higher risk. One easy approach to this problem might be to assume that the RR from Population 1 holds in Population 2: in this case, the risk

---

2. Reporting the stratified but imprecise results, however, may allow future researchers to pool across studies, as in a meta-analysis, to come up with better answers in important subgroups.

Table 6.2 AN ILLUSTRATION OF EFFECT MEASURE
MODIFICATION FOLLOWING A CHANGE IN BASELINE RISKS
FOR A NON-NULL EFFECT MEASURE.

Population 1	MI yes	MI no	Total	Risk
Exposed	400	1600	2000	0.250
Unexposed	250	1750	2000	0.125

Population 2	MI yes	MI no	Total	Risk
Exposed			3000	
Unexposed	750	2250	3000	0.250

among the exposed in Population 2 would be simply $0.250 \times 2 = 0.500$. If this was the case, however, the RD in Population 2 would be calculated as $0.500 - 0.250 = 0.250$—a number substantially different than in Population 1 (where RD = 0.125).

Alternatively, we might suppose that the RD from Population 1 holds in Population 2: in which case we would calculate the risk among the exposed in Population 2 as $0.250 + 0.125 = 0.375$. If this was the case, however, the RR in Population 2 would be calculated as $0.375/0.250 = 1.50$, a number substantially different from that of Population 1 (where RR = 2.0).

This leads us to a general rule here with three notes.

RULE

Specifically, if a baseline risk is different between two populations for a non-null association (1), then we will generally (2) have effect measure modification of either the RD or the RR, or both (3).

NOTES

1. If the effects in Population 1 had been null—for example, if the risk in the exposed and unexposed had been the same at 0.125—then no effect measure modification would be necessary. For example, in that case, the risk could be the same in both groups of Population 2, and the RD and RR would all be null in both populations.

2. This is a mathematical necessity in simple data; in real data we may (for example) have insufficient statistical power to distinguish such a phenomenon from chance. In addition, even when present, such effect measure modification may not be important.

3. EMM could be present on both scales at once. If in Population 2 the risk in the exposed were 0.75, the Population 2 RD would be 0.50 and the RR would be 3.0.

One implication of the necessity of effect measure modification after a change in baseline risk is that *any variable which causes the outcome is an EMM*: thus, any variable which has an arrow into the outcome on a DAG is an EMM on at least one measurement scale. As well, any variable merely *associated* with the outcome, for example through a backdoor path on a DAG, will typically also be an EMM (again on at least one scale). Thus, while DAGs cannot tell you that a variable is definitively an EMM for your current analysis, they can tell you which variables to consider as possible EMMs.

6.4.3 Most Confounders Are Modifiers

Historically, many epidemiologists have differentiated between confounding and effect measure modification by stating that confounding occurs when the stratum-specific estimates are largely equal (though are different from the crude, or overall, effect), whereas effect measure modification is when the stratum-specific estimates are quite different from each other.

As we explained earlier, however, for a non-null causal effect, any variable associated with a different risk of the outcome among the unexposed should be an EMM of either RD and RR (if not both). And all confounding variables (or, variables on open backdoor paths) meet this condition, either directly causing the outcome or through an association with the outcome. Thus, considering a confounding triangle such as Figure 6.5, we expect age to be an EMM of the effect of smoking on death on either the RD or RR scale (possibly both), unless the effect of smoking on death is null.

Since confounders are either direct or indirect causes of the outcome, or are associated with the outcome via an open backdoor path, we should therefore expect that most confounders also act as EMMs on at least one scale. For example, recall the data shown in Table 6.1, but now focus on the *ratio* rather than the difference scale: where $Z = 1$, the RR calculated from this table is 2.00. Where $Z = 0$, the RR is 1.33. This meets the description of effect measure modification on the ratio scale (the RRs are quite different between observed levels of Z) even though the causal structure shows confounding on all scales, and the data showed no effect measure modification on the RD scale. As such, we recommend against use of both the Mantel-Haenszel RD and RR approaches (see 6.6.1) in the same data because these approaches broadly assume constancy across strata of the confounder, and we should not expect constancy across strata of the confounder on both RD and RR at the same time.

This historically popular (though informal) definition of "confounder" as a variable for which the stratum-specific estimates are similar to each other but different from the crude (unadjusted) is thus shown to (often, though not always) be a definition *specific to the scale of the estimate* (RD vs. RR) rather than a *property of the causal structure itself* and therefore flawed. In contrast, DAGs are nonparametric and thus apply equally regardless of whether we are estimating an RD or RR. Thus, many variables we consider may be both confounders and EMMs simultaneously.

6.4.4 External Validity for Cohort Studies

The generalizability of a cohort study analysis to a specific target population works in a similar way to trials, although often we assume that an observational cohort study is more representative of a target population than a trial would be due to less stringent exclusion criteria. Briefly, ethical barriers to enrolling individuals into a cohort are generally lower than enrolling individuals into a trial simply because experimentation of any sort on humans, as in a trial, entails serious ethical considerations.

One key point to emphasize is that there are situations in which an observational study with uncontrolled confounding but good generalizability for a particular target population may have overall less bias *with respect to that target population* than a randomized trial with excellent internal validity (Westreich et al., 2019). In addition, you should note that EMMs are key in understanding external validity in a given target population: if the distribution of EMMs differs from your study sample to your target population, it is likely that the causal effect estimated in the study will be different from the causal effect you would have found if (counter to fact) the study had been performed directly in the target population. However, causal diagram approaches to generalizability also exist and may be more reliable than examining EMMs. In Chapter 9, we expand on the issues of generalizability and external validity more broadly, including describing simple quantitative methods for estimating the effects of observational and randomized studies in external target populations.

6.5 ADDITIONAL ISSUES IN OBSERVATIONAL COHORT STUDIES

6.5.1 Intention-to-Treat Analysis Versus Compliance-Corrected Analysis

As in randomized trials, a cohort study could be analyzed based on the exposure recorded at the first visit or based on the pattern of exposure over the course of follow-up, which can provide analogues to ITT and compliance-corrected analyses. In contrast to the randomized setting, however, an "ITT-type" analysis in an observational setting is subject to confounding, but dealing with confounding at a single time point is substantially easier in most cases than dealing with confounding of a time-varying exposure, which in general requires advanced methods not covered in this text (see Hernán & Robins, 2019, especially section 3).

6.5.2 Limitations and Cautions

Cohort studies, like randomized trials, can be limited in various ways. Earlier, we noted the potential limitations in terms of exchangeability and other causal identification conditions; here, we briefly address several more potential limitations.

Just as in a randomized trial, individuals enrolled in a cohort study can become *lost to follow-up*. Indeed, such losses may be more common in an observational setting exactly because the bar to entry and intensity of follow-up is lower than in a typical randomized trial. Regardless of incidence, such losses can bias results if they are not independent of the outcome (or made independent of the outcome analytically). And, as in randomized settings, right-censoring for administrative reasons is common though not likely to bias results.

Table 6.3 Two 2 × 2 tables for groups 0
and 1, with symbols instead of numbers
for generality

Group 0	Disease	No disease
Exposed	a_0	b_0
Unexposed	c_0	d_0
Group 1	**Disease**	**No disease**
Exposed	a_1	b_1
Unexposed	c_1	d_1

A randomized trial typically serves to investigate the effect of a treatment or intervention—something we can actually do. In contrast, observational studies in epidemiology often estimate the effects of exposures rather than the effects of interventions to remove those exposures. So an observational study might examine the exposure of smoking, while a trial would be unlikely (for ethical reasons, if no other) to randomized smoking but could instead randomize a smoking cessation intervention. One additional caution is in order relating to the "Table 2 Fallacy" (Box 6.2 and Table 6.3).

6.6 ANALYTIC APPROACHES TO OBSERVATIONAL COHORT DATA

The analytic methods we addressed in the previous chapter can be applied to observational cohort data just as they can to data from randomized trials; however, the presence of confounding means that interpreting the results of such methods is far more complicated. Thus, in this section, we will concentrate on introducing the fundamentals of how to use both Mantel-Haenszel and IPW approaches to control confounding. We will also go into additional detail about how regression works.

At least some material in this section relies on a general framework for confounded data in two categories. A general (symbolic) 2 × 2 × 2 table is used, with letters (subscripted for group number) instead of numbers for each cell. Of course, the actual letters might vary in other presentations of such tables, as might the table set-up (e.g., outcome might be on the rows, and exposure on the columns).

6.6.1 Mantel-Haenszel Estimators

As noted earlier, a key method for estimating a single unconfounded effect of an exposure on a disease is the Mantel-Haenszel estimator.[3] For two strata (0,1) and two general 2 × 2 tables, as shown in Table 6.3, we can estimate the Mantel-Haenszel RD (RD_{MH}) with the following formula (Cochran, 1954; Rothman,

---

3. These estimators are sometimes called Cochran-Mantel-Haenszel estimators; however, the Cochran-Mantel-Haenszel is the name of the statistical test associated with the following methods, not the method itself.

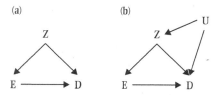

Figure 6.6 (a) Simple confounding triangle. (b) Elaborated confounding structure.

Greenland, & Lash, 2008), where z indicates level of confounder, such that $\sum_z f_z$ means "sum f over strata of z," and $n_z = a_z + b_z + c_z + d_z$.

$$\widehat{RD}_{mh} = \frac{\sum_z \{RD_z w_z\}}{\sum_z w_z}, \quad \text{where } w_z = (a_z + b_z)(c_z + d_z)/n_z$$

Recall that Mantel-Haenszel approaches are a means of combining stratum-specific estimates; these methods are expected to work in a closed cohort (Chapter 1) with no losses to follow-up. Note how the quantity shown in the formula is a weighted average of the effects in the two strata. Here, we rewrite this formula to make this weighting clearer for a case where we have only two groups:

$$\widehat{RD}_{mh} = \frac{RD_0 w_0 + RD_1 w_1}{w_0 + w_1}$$

Now we apply this formula to sample data. Figure 6.6a shows a simple confounding triangle (similar to Figure 6.3; Figure 6.6b shows a slightly different confounding structure which will become relevant later in this chapter). Table 6.4 shows data consistent with Figure 6.6a. First, suppose that the outcome is measured at a set time (say, 1 year after start of study) for all participants. Second, note that the data in Table 6.4 are consistent with the arrow from Z to E because the probability of exposure differs by level of Z ($2,500/(2,500 + 750) \neq 1,000/(1,000 + 1,500)$). Likewise note that the arrow from Z to D is shown in that the overall (total) risk of D likewise differs by level of Z ($0.231 \neq 0.124$). The arrow from E to D indicates that we hypothesize a true causal effect of E on D: here, shown by the causal effect of exposure on disease D among $Z = 0$ ($0.24 - 0.20 = 0.04$) and $Z = 1$ ($0.16 - 0.10 = 0.06$). That crude RD is higher than both of these stratum specific estimates ($0.217 - 0.133 = 0.084$) is consistent with confounding by Z.

If we apply the preceding formula to the data in Table 6.4, we get weights as follows:

$$w_0 = \frac{(a_0 + b_0)(c_0 + d_0)}{n_0} = \frac{(600 + 1900)(150 + 600)}{3250} = 576.923$$

$$w_1 = \frac{(a_1 + b_1)(c_1 + d_1)}{n_1} = \frac{(160 + 840)(150 + 1350)}{2500} = 600.000$$

and so

$$\widehat{RD}_{mh} = \frac{RD_0 w_0 + RD_1 w_1}{w_0 + w_1} = \frac{0.04 \times 576.923 + 0.06 \times 600}{576.923 + 600} = 0.050$$

This makes sense, in that we expect a weighted average of 0.04 and 0.06 to fall in between those two. If we weight the two estimates approximately the same, we should indeed expect to come up with a number right in the range of 0.05. Test your own intuition: If we reapply the same method with the same group of $Z = 1$, but only 10% of those observed in $Z = 0$ (so that in $Z = 0$, {a,b,c,d} = {60, 190, 15, 60}), would the RD_{MH} be closer to RD_0 or RD_1? (Try this and see!)

The Mantel-Haenszel RR can be estimated similarly (Nurminen, 1981; Rothman et al., 2008). Using the same weights as the Mantel-Haenszel RD, specifically

$$w_z = (a_z + b_z)(c_z + d_z)/n_z$$

we can calculate the Mantel-Haenszel RR as follows, where $R_{E=1,z}$ is the risk among the exposed for some level of z, and $R_{E=0,z}$ is defined likewise.[4]

$$\widehat{RR}_{mh} = \frac{\sum_z R_{E=1,z} w_z}{\sum_z R_{E=0,z} w_z} = \frac{\sum_z \dfrac{a_z(c_z + d_z)}{n_z}}{\sum_z \dfrac{c_z(a_z + b_z)}{n_z}}$$

Table 6.4 DATA CONSISTENT WITH THE DIRECTED ACYCLIC GRAPH (DAG) IN FIGURE 6.6(A)

Z = 0 only	D yes	D no	Total	Risk
Exposed	600	1,900	2,500	0.240
Unexposed	150	600	N750	0.200
Total	750	2,500	3,250	0.231
Z = 1 only	**D yes**	**D no**	**Total**	**Risk**
Exposed	160	840	1,000	0.160
Unexposed	150	1,350	1,500	0.100
Total	310	2,190	2,500	0.124
All Z	**D yes**	**D no**	**Total**	**Risk**
Exposed	760	2,740	3,500	0.217
Unexposed	300	1,950	2,250	0.133
Total	1,060	4,690	5,750	0.184

---

4. There is also a Mantel-Haenszel odds ratio; this is given in Chapter 7.

Recall that Mantel-Haenszel approaches typically assume that the effect estimates being combined across strata are roughly equal. As we noted earlier, because most confounders are also EMMs on at least one scale, we may wish to avoid applying Mantel-Haenszel approaches to estimate both the RD and RR for the same data. A similar caution applies to any method which assumes constancy of effect measure by strata.

6.6.2 Inverse Probability Weights

The IPW itself is the reciprocal of the probability that an individual has the exposure they have, given the value of their covariate. That's a mouthful, so we'll write it out in a formula:

$$IPW_{Z=z} = \frac{1}{Pr(E = e \mid Z = z)}$$

What does that formula mean? Again considering the data in Table 6.4 (and replicated on the left side of Table 6.5), we would calculate an IPW for $Z = 0$ as the inverse of the probability of exposure (or nonexposure) at a given level of Z. Among $Z = 0$, the probability of exposure is 2,500/3,250, or 0.769; the weight for the exposed is therefore the inverse, $1/0.769 = 1.30$. A calculation for the unexposed yields a probability of 750/3,250, or 0.231; the weight is $1/0.231 = 4.33$. Similar calculations for $Z = 1$ gives us weights of 2.5 and 1.67 for the exposed and unexposed groups, respectively. In practice, weights are often estimated not from tables but with regression models (Cole & Hernán, 2008) and increasingly with machine learning approaches.

How do we use these weights? We apply these weights (in Table 6.5) row-by-row: each individual cell (a, b, c, d) is multiplied by the weight for its row. For

Table 6.5 APPLYING INVERSE PROBABILITY OF TREATMENT WEIGHTS TO THE DATA IN TABLE 6.4

		Raw data				IPW	Weighted data			
		D yes	D no	Total	Risk		D yes	D no	Total	Risk
Z = 0	Exposed	600	1,900	2,500	0.240	1.30	780	2,470	3,250	
	Unexposed	150	600	750	0.200	4.33	650	2,600	3,250	
Z = 1	Exposed	160	840	1,000	0.160	2.50	400	2,100	2,500	
	Unexposed	150	1,350	1,500	0.100	1.67	250	2,250	2,500	
All Z	Exposed	760	2,740	3,500	0.217		1,180	4,570	5,750	0.205
	Unexposed	300	1,950	2,250	0.133		900	4,850	5,750	0.157
	Total	1,060	4,690	5,750	0.184					

example, 600 (box a in $Z = 0$) is multiplied by 1.30 to yield 780. Similarly 150 (box c in $Z = 0$) is multiplied by 4.33 to yield 650. Thus, we fill out two new, *weighted* 2×2 tables. Note that after applying the weights, the total number of exposed and unexposed individuals is the same in each of the $Z = 0$ and $Z = 1$ groups: in $Z = 0$ there are 3,250 weighted exposed individuals and 3,250 weighted unexposed individuals. In $Z = 1$ those numbers are both 2,500.

Earlier, we noted that the arrow from Z to E was shown by the fact that the probability of E differed by level of Z in the raw data. But in the reweighted data, the probability of exposure is the same at both levels of Z: 50% of those at $Z = 0$ are exposed, as are 50% of those at $Z = 1$. This is consistent with a new DAG, in which the weighting has effectively removed the $Z{\rightarrow}E$ arrow *in the weighted data* (Figure 6.7).

If there is no $Z{\rightarrow}E$ arrow, there is no open backdoor path from E to D; thus, we can conclude that the reweighted data are in fact free of confounding by Z. Therefore, we can proceed by simply taking reweighted data in the two strata and recombining the strata into a single 2×2 table (the crude 2×2 table for the weighted *pseudo-population*), in Table 6.5. In this last 2×2 table, we can simply determine risks and compare them, finding a weighted RD of 0.049 and a weighted RR of 1.311. This is a slightly different estimate from what was found using the Mantel-Haenszel approach earlier; both are weighted averages, but they use different weights.

IPWs are a broadly useful approach to dealing with potential biases in analysis, and have been applied to deal not only with confounding (Cole & Hernán, 2008) but also with missing data (Seaman & White, 2013) and external validity (Cole & Stuart, 2010). As an example of the versatility of this approach, we offer this: if it is true that exposure and confounder(s) are not associated in a weighted pseudo-population, it follows that analyses—including figures—deriving from that pseudo-population will be free of those same measured confounders (assuming correct model specification) (Cole & Hernán, 2004). Thus, once we calculate IPWs and use them to reweight our data into a pseudo-population, we are free to draw crude survival curves in that pseudo-population, and we can interpret them free of concerns of confounding by measured variables (assuming we have calculated the weights correctly; and, of course, not free of confounding by unmeasured variables).

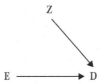

Figure 6.7 Directed acyclic graph illustrating the effect of inverse probability weighting on Figure 6.6a.

6.6.3 Regression Analysis

In real data, there are often numerous confounding variables (or confounding variables are continuous rather than dichotomous; i.e., "age in months" rather than "age above or below 36 months"): in such cases, tabular approaches will often not be viable. Regression analysis is a key popular alternative, and we will give some bare rudiments of this approach to data here.

Regression analysis is not entirely dissimilar to middle school math in which you learned that a line can be defined as $Y = mX + b$, where Y is the outcome (dependent) variable, X is the exposure (independent) variable, b is the intercept (the Y value when $X = 0$), and m is the slope (the change in y per unit increase in X). An equivalent regression might be stated as

$$Y = \beta_0 + \beta_1 X + \epsilon$$

or, alternatively,

$$E(Y) = \beta_0 + \beta_1 X$$

where (m, b) are equivalent to (β_1, β_0), $E(Y)$ indicates the statistical expectation of Y (which equals to the probability that $Y = 1$ when Y is dichotomous), and the expectation term allows us to drop the error term in the second equation. As this implies, regression analysis is similar to the "two points make a line" math lessons from your youth—though it is somewhat more complicated.

Several key issues are worth calling out. First, in regression analysis, you typically have more than two data points and thus (near universally) you cannot draw a single line through all data points. Instead, the task of fitting a regression model to the data is minimizing error between the regression line you define (by defining the equivalents of m and b in the middle school math equation) and the observed data. How error is calculated and minimized varies, but using *sum of squared error* (as in ordinary least squares) is perhaps the most common approach. Regression approaches typically require you to make assumptions (or assertions!) about the distribution of the errors in the analysis. Finally, in regression analysis, you likewise typically have more than two variables.

We illustrate this with the example applied to the data in Table 6.4. One regression model for these data ignoring Z is

$$E(D) = \Pr(D) = \beta_0 + \beta_1 E,$$

which we would apply to the data in Table 6.4. Because this equation omits any Z term, it implicitly fits only to the data for "All Z" in the table. We can estimate the beta coefficients for this model as follows from the raw data among "All Z": When E is equal to 0, what is the risk of D? From the table, we can read off

"0.133," and thus this is the value of β_0. Given this value, when $\beta_1 = 1$ we can rewrite the preceding equation as $\Pr(D) = 0.133 + \beta_1 \times 1 = 0.133 + \beta_1$; since we know from Table 6.4 that the probability of D when $E = 1$ is 0.217, we can calculate $\beta_1 = 0.217 - 0.133 = 0.084$. (Reminder: in real data, things are rarely this simple! And, as well, many epidemiologists object strongly to modeling a binary outcome with a linear model, among other reasons because it can predict values outside of the range of the data.)

Not coincidentally, this is exactly the same calculation for the crude RD: in such a (simplified!) regression approach, the coefficient attached to the exposure variable (in this case β_1) can often be interpreted as the RD. However, that RD cannot always be interpreted causally, as in this case, where we know that there is confounding of the $E{\to}D$ relationship by Z (Figure 6.6a). If we want a causal interpretation of β_1, we must fit a regression equation that accounts for potential confounding by Z, for example:

$$E(D) = \Pr(D) = \beta_0 + \beta_1 E + \beta_2 Z.$$

Again, because these data are simple, we can proceed as we did earlier. Now, β_0 is the probability of D when E and Z are both equal to 0: from the $Z = 0$ stratum in Table 6.4, this value is 0.200. We can then simply think of the value of Z as the change in the probability of D when Z moves from 0 to 1. Since the risk in the unexposed among those with $Z = 1$ is equal to 0.100, the change from 0.200 is −0.100. Thus, $\beta_2 = -0.100$. Now for β_1: when $Z = 0$, the change in probability of D associated with a one-unit increase in E is the $Z = 0$ RD, 0.04. This implies that β_1 should equal 0.04. When $Z = 1$, the change in probability of D associated with a one-unit increase in E is the $Z = 1$ RD, 0.06. This implies that that β_1 should equal 0.06. Since β_1 cannot equal 0.04 and 0.06 simultaneously, we must (again!) pick some point between 0.04 and 0.06—one which minimizes the sum of squared-errors.

This last step is not trivial by hand, so we have used a computer program instead which gives us a value of $\beta_1 = 0.0502$ (and, incidentally, gives us slightly different estimated value for $\beta_0 = 0.1922$; this change is due to the inclusion of Z in the model). This estimate for β_1 could be interpreted as "the 1-year RD comparing exposed to unexposed individuals while holding Z constant at any level" or alternatively "while adjusting for Z." In collapsing across levels of Z, we are imposing a modeling assumption that the effect is the same in both levels of Z—and therefore that we can use the evidence from both groups to estimate a single effect size.

There are multiple different types of regression, many of which produce measures other than the RD: one popular option is *logistic regression*, which produces odds ratios (specifically, it produces beta coefficients as in our preceding examples; we then raise e [i.e., 2.71828 . . .] to the power of the beta coefficient corresponding to the exposure to yield an odds ratio comparing the two exposure categories). All types of regression typically require strong assumptions about the shape of the relationship between the exposure, covariates/confounders, and the outcome; the reader can find numerous textbooks elaborating on these topics (Can—and should!) Regression is an extremely common technique for dealing with epidemiologic data, and the reader who wishes to contribute or even just understand the epidemiologic literature would be well-advised to understand regression.

6.7 SUMMARY

Prospective observational cohort studies are a mainstay of epidemiologic research and have both advantages and disadvantages for assessing causal effects of exposures compared to other study designs, particularly randomized trials. On the positive side, they are often highly representative of intended target populations, can be larger in enrollment and longer in duration than randomized trials, and are more realistic in many ways than randomized studies. On the negative side, observational cohort studies can suffer from uncontrolled confounding and large treatment variation, and they may have more potential for measurement error because of the way they are conducted in practice.

We compare these two designs further in future chapters. In the next chapter, we describe case-control studies, which are perhaps most productively thought of as cohort studies with an added step of sampling based on outcome status.

6.8 NOTES ON REVIEWING A PUBLISHED OBSERVATIONAL COHORT STUDY

For the reader of the observational literature, reviewing an observational cohort study can be tricky. Several points worth considering, and implied from the preceding material, include:

1. Is there a hypothetical (or real-world) equivalent randomized trial to this cohort study, and, if so, what would such a trial look like? Asking this question can help us clarify whether the analytic methods for this study are appropriate and whether particular analytic decisions are consistent with the data.
2. Closely related to the first point, what are the treatments/exposures and outcomes?
3. Does this study attempt to show a causal effect? Authors frequently state that they are interested only in finding associations, but if they control for covariates, or particularly "confounders" in multivariable regression models, then their implicit aim is generally to estimate causal effects, not associations per se. If the authors are trying to estimate a causal effect, make sure to consider whether there might be uncontrolled confounding—but also consider issues of selection bias and relation of the study sample to the target population (if a target population can even be identified clearly from the work).

4. In addition to issues of confounding, treatment variation is a common issue in interpreting causal effects in observational settings: Is there meaningful treatment variation at play? Note that under many circumstances a wide range of treatment versions is consistent with a more broadly defined exposure or exposure assignment. Consider an observational study of statins in which dose and regularity of taking statins differs immensely among ever-users of statins. Such treatment variation may prevent the paper from making conclusions about the effect of statins on a specific outcome. On the other hand, it might in such a case be more defensible to try to estimate the effect of a potential policy assigning patients to take statins since the causal effect of a policy would include a variety of ways in which statins were taken.

5. Is the exposure under study time-varying? If so, did the authors deal with this situation using the correct methods (which are beyond the scope of this book; see Hernán & Robins, 2019)?

6. Were the exposure, outcome, and confounders measured accurately? What were the sensitivity and specificity of the measurement tools used to measure these variables? What steps were taken, if any, to ensure accurate measurement? What steps were taken, if any, to analyze the impact of inaccurate measurement?

REFERENCES

Cochran, W. G. (1954). Some methods for strengthening common chi-square tests. *Biometrics, 10*, 417–451.

Cole, S. R., & Hernán, M. A. (2004). Adjusted survival curves with inverse probability weights. *Computer Methods and Programs in Biomedicine, 75*(1), 45–49.

Cole, S. R., & Hernán, M. A. (2008). Constructing inverse probability weights for marginal structural models. *American Journal of Epidemiology, 168*(6), 656–664.

Cole, S. R., & Stuart, E. A. (2010). Generalizing evidence from randomized clinical trials to target populations: The ACTG 320 trial. *American Journal of Epidemiology, 172*(1), 107–115. doi:kwq084 [pii]10.1093/aje/kwq084

Hernán, M. A., & Robins, J. M. (2019). *Causal inference.* Boca Raton: Chapman & Hall/CRC. Retrieved from http://www.hsph.harvard.edu/miguel-hernan/causal-inference-book/.

Joffe, M. M., & Rosenbaum, P. R. (1999). Invited commentary: Propensity scores. *American Journal of Epidemiology, 150*(4), 327–333.

Nurminen, M. (1981). Asymptotic efficiency of general noniterative estimators of common relative risk. *Biometrika, 68*(2), 525–530.

Rehkopf, D. H., Glymour, M. M., & Osypuk, T. L. (2016). The consistency assumption for causal inference in social epidemiology: When a rose is not a rose. *Current Epidemiology Reports, 3*(1), 63–71. doi:10.1007/s40471-016-0069-5

Rosenbaum, P. R., & Rubin, D. B. (1983). The central role of the propensity score in observational studies for causal effects. *Biometrika, 70*(1), 41–55.

Rothman, K. J., Greenland, S., & Lash, T. L. (2008). *Modern epidemiology* (3rd ed.). Philadelphia: Lippincott Williams & Wilkins.

Seaman, S. R., & White, I. R. (2013). Review of inverse probability weighting for dealing with missing data. *Statistical Methods in Medical Research, 22*(3), 278–295. doi:10.1177/0962280210395740

VanderWeele, T. J. (2009). On the distinction between interaction and effect modification. *Epidemiology, 20*(6), 863–871. doi:10.1097/EDE.0b013e3181ba333c

VanderWeele, T. J., & Robinson, W. R. (2014). On the causal interpretation of race in regressions adjusting for confounding and mediating variables. *Epidemiology, 25*(4), 473–484. doi:10.1097/EDE.0000000000000105

Westreich, D., Edwards, J. K., Lesko, C. R., Cole, S. R., & Stuart, E. A. (2019). Target validity and the hierarchy of study designs. *American Journal of Epidemiology, 188*(2), 438–443. doi:10.1093/aje/kwy228

Westreich, D., & Greenland, S. (2013). The table 2 fallacy: Presenting and interpreting confounder and modifier coefficients. *American Journal of Epidemiology, 177*(4), 292–298. doi:10.1093/aje/kws412

7

Case-Control Studies

In contrast to an observational cohort study in which participants are identified, exposures are measured, and then outcomes status is measured after follow-up, a case-control study is an observational study in which we sample participants based on their outcome status, often only after all outcomes have already occurred.

Take our previous example of a fictional vaccine to prevent heart attack. In a randomized trial (Chapter 5), we might flip a coin to assign some participants to receive the vaccine and others to receive a placebo (and hope that participants were highly adherent to their treatment assignment). In a prospective observational cohort study (Chapter 6), we could allow participants to choose on their own to receive the vaccine or no vaccine. In both cases, we follow participants over time to see who might experience a heart attack by the end of our study period—perhaps for 5 years.

In a case-control study, by contrast, we might start by identifying individuals who had experienced heart attacks in a given span of time (cases), say within the last 5 years. We would gather information about those individuals' exposure to the vaccine 5 years ago. Then, we might identify individuals who had *not* had heart attacks in that same span of time (controls). Since the purpose of these control subjects is to represent the background levels of exposure to vaccine, we would then gather information about their exposure to the vaccine, similarly 5 years ago. We could then analyze the resulting data.

This somewhat abstract description of a case-control study may be difficult to understand. It is easier to build intuition around case-control studies by starting with a prospective observational cohort study and then describing how a case-control study can be seen as a particular way of sampling from the data of the cohort study, using real numbers. Such an exercise is key to understanding this design, in fact. Case-control studies are often perceived as inferior to observational cohort studies—in particular, because the identification of outcomes *before* exposures are measured leads to concerns about biased exposure assessment and because of concerns around selection bias in selection of controls. These concerns are reasonable in some case-control designs. However, as we will see, such global guidance to view results from case-control studies as an inferior source of evidence is likely misguided. As we will discuss, case-control studies can always be thought of as implicitly (and sometimes explicitly) nested in a cohort; especially

Epidemiology by Design: A Causal Approach to the Health Sciences. Daniel Westreich, Oxford University Press (2020). © Oxford University Press.
DOI: 10.1093/oso/9780190665760.001.0001

Table 7.1 TRUE RELATIONSHIP BETWEEN PRESENCE
OF A PRO-INFLAMMATORY GENETIC MARKER G AND
5-YEAR RISK OF HEART ATTACK

Full data	MI yes	MI no	Total	Risk
G yes	200	1,800	2,000	0.100
G no	100	1,900	2,000	0.050
Total	300	3,700	4,000	0.075

in the explicit case, exposure information may be straightforward to collect from the underlying cohort.

Invented in the 19th century, it is widely accepted that the first modern case-control study can be credited to Dr. Janet Lane-Claypon, in a 1926 study which was perhaps the first to find an association between reproductive history and risk of breast cancer in women (Lane-Claypon, 1926; Paneth, Susser, & Susser, 2002a, 2002b).

7.1 SAMPLING FROM A COHORT STUDY

Consider a prospective observational cohort study of 4,000 participants followed for 5 years for the outcome of heart attack. At the beginning of the study, we take a blood sample from each participant and store that sample (in deep freeze) for the duration of the study. After the completion of the study, a new pro-inflammatory single nucleotide polymorphism G is discovered; we suspect that having G might increase risk of heart attack (myocardial infarction, or MI). The *unobserved* true levels of the exposure of the genetic marker and outcomes are shown in the 2 × 2 table in Table 7.1; we assume there is no confounding of the relationship shown in this table. From Table 7.1, we calculate the true risk of MI in the exposed (study participants *with* G) of 10% and in the unexposed (study participants *without* G) of 5%. The true risk difference is therefore 5%, the true risk ratio is 2.00, and the true odds ratio (OR) is 2.11.

Suppose further that, due to limited funds, we are not able to test every individual for G. In fact, we only have sufficient funds to test 600 blood samples. How shall we decide who to test?

There are many possible answers to this question. Perhaps the most obvious answer is "take a random sample of 600 of the 4,000 individuals and test them." Under simple random sampling, the expected risks will be the same (Table 7.2) in

Table 7.2 DATA FROM TABLE 7.1 UNDER SIMPLE RANDOM
SAMPLING (WHERE PROBABILITY OF SELECTION IS 15%)

Sampled data	MI yes (sampled)	MI no (sampled)	Total	Risk
G yes	30	270	300	0.100
G no	15	285	300	0.050
Total	45	575	600	0.075

Table 7.3 A GENERIC 2 × 2 TABLE

Exposure	Outcome	
	Yes	No
Yes	a	b
No	c	d

each case, and contrasts of risks that we calculate will be unbiased (e.g., the risk ratio from Table 7.2 remains 2.00, the OR remains 2.11).

However, this approach may be suboptimal in terms of *variance*. We have not discussed variance much in this book thus far, but here introducing a basic variance calculation will be helpful in understanding our sampling approach. Given a generic (symbolic) 2 × 2 table shown in Table 7.3, we know from previous chapters that we can calculate the OR from this table as

$$OR = ad / bc$$

The variance of the natural log of the OR is:

$$Var(\text{In}(OR)) = \frac{1}{a} + \frac{1}{b} + \frac{1}{c} + \frac{1}{d}$$

and therefore the standard error of the natural log of the OR is

$$SE(\text{In}(OR)) = \sqrt{\frac{1}{a} + \frac{1}{b} + \frac{1}{c} + \frac{1}{d}}$$

Thus, from Table 7.1, we would calculate an OR and 95% confidence interval (CI) of 2.11 (1.65, 2.71) (full details shown in Section 7.5) and the variance of the natural log of the OR (var(ln(OR))) is 0.016. From Table 7.2, we would use the same calculation to find an OR of 2.11 (95% CI 1.11, 4.01) and a var(ln(OR)) of 0.107.

The variance calculated from Table 7.2 is about 10 times the variance calculated from Table 7.1. That is a large increase in variance, or in the width of CIs. In examining the equation for variance just given, we can quickly see why. The *largest* terms in the variance equation are those in which the denominator is *smallest*. For example, the components of the variance for the data shown in Table 7.2 are 1/30, 1/270, 1/15, and 1/285. Thus, the largest components are driven by the smallest cells, a and c. Cells a and c are the smallest because (i) heart attacks are relatively rare in the original population (only 7.5% incidence total) and we sampled few people in total (only 600).

This leads us to ask: Could we have chosen a different group of 600 people to analyze, still have obtained an unbiased estimate of effect, but not increased our variance as much? Intuition immediately suggests that we would need to

Table 7.4 DATA FROM TABLE 7.1 UNDER SAMPLING
WHERE WE START BY TAKING ALL THOSE
WHO EXPERIENCED THE OUTCOME

	MI yes (complete)	. . .	Total	Risk
G yes	200			
G no	100			
Total	300		600	0.50

Note that the column labeled " . . . " is explained in the text.

ensure that *a* and *c* are larger: one immediate possibility is to consider taking all 300 people who experienced heart attack (MI) into our new study, for testing for genotype G. Note that when we do this it may look as if the risk in the total population is distorted: instead of being 7.5%, as in the original cohort, that risk is now 50% in our sample for this study. This is shown in Table 7.4; you may notice that in this table we have deliberately omitted the name of the third column, which is " . . . " in the figure rather than "MI no (sampled)") as in Table 7.2. We explain later.

A next step might be to fill in the remaining column with 300 people who did *not* experience MI during follow-up: of the 3,700 people who met this definition in the original study, 1,800 had G yes, and so we would expect $\frac{1800}{3700} \times 300 \approx 146$

to have G and $\frac{1900}{3700} \times 300 \approx 154$ (or 300 − 146) to not have G (we ignore decimals for convenience). If we take this resulting 2 × 2 table and calculate risks from it, we immediately see serious problems: the risk among those with G in Table 7.5 is 57.8%, dramatically different from the 10% found in the original table. Likewise, the risk in those without G in Table 7.5 is 39.4%, not at all the 5% seen in the original. As noted earlier, the overall risk is also wrong. The risk difference is 18.4% (not 10%) and the risk ratio is 1.47 (not 2.00).

Table 7.5 DATA WHEN WE EXTEND TABLE 7.4
TO INCLUDE 300 INDIVIDUALS WHO DID *NOT*
HAVE HEART ATTACK

	MI yes (complete)	. . .	Total	Risk
G yes	200	146	346	0.578
G no	100	154	254	0.394
Total	300	300	600	0.500

Note that the column labeled " . . . " is explained in the text.

The OR, calculated as $\dfrac{ad}{bc} = \dfrac{200 \times 154}{146 \times 100} = 2.1095890$ or approximately 2.11. Which—contrary to the risks and the risk difference and ratios—is (more or less) identical to what we saw in the original data. This finding may be unexpected to readers who have not traveled this path before! This is a first example of a case-control study, and if we calculate our 95% CIs and variance for this study, we find 2.11 (95% CI 1.52, 2.93) and a variance of 0.028, which is far closer to the variance in the total sample (Table 7.1, 0.016) than in the simple random sample (Table 7.2, 0.107).

Now, let's consider an additional approach, one where we again start by taking all the cases as in Table 7.4. Now, rather than selecting the remaining 300 individuals from those who did not experience a heart attack during follow-up (as we did in Table 7.5), we instead choose those individuals from among the 4,000 individuals who were *present at the baseline of the cohort study*. Since half the cohort had G and half did not at baseline, we would expect 150 individuals in each exposure group (150 G yes, 150 G no; see Table 7.6). If we calculate the risks, risk differences, and risk ratios from this table, we will again find that we are wrong compared to the original cohort results: these calculations are left as an exercise for you. Calculating the OR, however, as

$$\frac{ad}{bc} = \frac{200 \times 150}{150 \times 100} = 2.00$$

we find that it is exactly equal to the *risk ratio* in the original cohort (from Table 7.1). We omit variance calculations here (they are quite similar as those for Table 7.5) and challenge you instead to consider why this sampling from those present at baseline leads our case-control OR to mimic the cohort risk ratio of 2.00, while sampling from those who did *not* experience the outcome, as in Table 7.5, leads our case-control OR to mimic the cohort OR of 2.11.

7.2 CASE-CONTROL STUDIES

Both Table 7.5 and Table 7.6 show the results of *case-control studies*, nested inside of the cohort shown in Table 7.1. In both Tables 7.5 and 7.6, we study all cases

Table 7.6 Data when we extend Table 7.4 to include 300 individuals selected from cohort *at baseline*

	MI yes (complete)	. . .	Total	Risk
G yes	200	150	350	0.571
G no	100	150	250	0.400
Total	300	300	600	0.500

Note that the column labeled " . . . " is explained in the text.

Table 7.7 GENERAL 2 × 2 TABLE SCHEMA FOR A COHORT STUDY (LEFT) AND
A CASE-CONTROL STUDY (RIGHT)

Cohort study	Outcome		Total	Case-control study		
	Yes	No			Cases	Controls
Exposed	A	B	A + B	Exposed	a	b
Not exposed	C	D	C + D	Not exposed	c	d
Total	A + C	B + D	N				n

of disease (the cases) and a sample of non-cases (the controls). Depending on how we sample those controls, the OR from the case-control study (which we will hereafter refer to as the *case-control OR* or *ccOR*) can serve to estimate either the cohort OR (Table 7.5) or the cohort risk ratio (Table 7.6). We discuss the purpose of controls and various approaches to control sampling further later.

Table 7.7 shows a general 2 × 2 schema for a prospective observational cohort study (left) and a case-control study (right), the latter regardless of the manner in which controls are sampled.

Note that, by convention, we do not give "Total" columns in the case-control study because (as we illustrated earlier) the sampling process for a case-control study dramatically distorts the denominators, making the direct calculation of risks untenable. Relatedly, as implied by Table 7.7, the empty column heading in Tables 7.4–7.6 should read "Controls," and the columns labeled "MI yes (complete)" would be better labeled as "Cases." We will label according to the Table 7.7 schema from this point forward.

7.2.1 Why Do We Conduct Case-Control Studies?

We conduct case-control studies because they are an efficient way of estimating both measures (of association and effect) as well as variances, similar to those obtained in a cohort study. By "efficient," here, we mean that case-control studies may be both faster in time and less expensive to conduct than alternatives. In the example we described, we were constrained by money: we could only afford to run 600 tests; the case-control studies showed a substantial gain in efficiency compared to choosing 600 people completely at random from the underlying data. Again, in the preceding example, the variance of the log-OR in the full data (Table 7.1) was 0.016, and the variance for the log-OR in a random 10% sample was 0.107. In a case-control sample using all the cases and an equal number of controls (1:1 case-control sampling), the variance of the log-OR was 0.028. Case-control samples using all the cases and 2, 3, or 4 controls per case (1:2, 1:3, 1:4 sampling) would have variances of 0.021, 0.019, and 0.018, respectively (although, of course, they would require us to use more blood tests, and so be less resource-efficient). See also Box 7.1.

Box 7.1

How Many Controls per Case?

It is notable that, at least in this case, the gain from a random 10% sample to a
1:1 case-control match is quite large (from 0.107 to 0.028), but after that point
adding another 300 controls has a relatively small impact on variance (from 0.028
to 0.021). It is broadly thought and widely repeated that the case-control sampling
ratio of 1:4 is the point of diminishing returns in terms of variance, but it is unclear how widely this recommendation holds empirically.

The second type of efficiency that case-control studies can provide arises in
time. Consider a pressing health question about a rare outcome, for example
a particular cancer. Accumulating sufficient numbers of a very rare outcome
requires either very long follow-up time, enormous numbers of participants, or
both. In contrast, many US states and many national health systems maintain
cancer registries that record every cancer diagnosed within that region. We might
be able to address a question about the cancer efficiently in time (and resources)
by finding all cases of the cancer over a particular time period (1990–2010), which
would allow us to fill in one of the columns of our 2 × 2 table. Then we have to
identify our controls to fill in the rest of the table.

7.2.2 Identifying Controls

The purpose of controls in a typical (unmatched) case-control study is to represent the source population from which the cases arose, and in particular the
distribution of *exposure and confounders in the source population from which the
cases arose*. This is a relatively easy thing to do if the source population being
considered is an actual cohort study, as in our example. However, it may be more
difficult if the case-control study in question is nested inside a cohort only in a
conceptual sense.

For example, considering a case-control study based in a cancer registry (as
just described), there is no explicit cohort study inside of which the cancer registry is nested: the registry has captured not all cancer cases in, say, a prospective
observational cohort study—but rather in a state. Still, considering which *implicit
cohort* the case-control study is nested inside can be useful in considering what
controls are appropriate. In the case of a cancer registry for North Carolina, anyone living in North Carolina from 1990 to 2010 who was diagnosed with cancer
is included in the registry; thus, one possible (narrow) description of the population from which the cases arose might be "all those living in North Carolina in
1990 who remained living in the state until 2010." While that population might
be difficult to identify, it should be at least conceptually clear to you how the cases
arose from that population.

Table 7.8 A COHORT STUDY SCHEMA WITH CALCULATIONS OF RISKS, RISK RATIOS,
ODDS, AND ODDS RATIOS (ORs)

Cohort study	Outcome		Total	Risk	Risk ratio	Odds	OR
	Yes	No					
Exposed	A	B	$A + B$	$A/(A + B)$	$(A/(A + B))\,/$	A/B	$AD\,/\,BC$
Not exposed	C	D	$C + D$	$C/(C + D)$	$(C/(C + D))$	C/D	
Total	$A + C$	$B + D$					

7.2.3 Types of Sampling

There are three main ways to sample controls that we will discuss here: cumulative sampling, case-cohort sampling, and incidence density sampling. To explain the first two, we extend the left panel of Table 7.7 into Table 7.8, where we can calculate the risks, risk ratio, odds, and OR symbolically.

7.2.3.1 CUMULATIVE CONTROL SAMPLING

Cumulative sampling (sometimes *cumulative incidence sampling*) occurs when we sample controls from among the *non-cases at the end of follow-up*, without regard to their true exposure status; the results of *cumulative sampling* were shown in Table 7.5. When we use cumulative sampling, the resulting ccOR will in general estimate the cohort OR.

Why should this be? Consider a case-control study sampled from the cohort study in Table 7.8; we show the schema for this case-control study in Table 7.9. First we take all the cases, so that the number of exposed cases $a = A$ and the number of unexposed cases $c = C$. Then we turn to control sampling. Cumulative sampling of controls considers only a sample (g, where $0 < g < 1$) of the non-cases (B and D) independent of exposure status. This means that our exposed controls $b = gB$ are a fraction of the exposed non-outcomes from the cohort, and our unexposed controls $d = gD$, the same fraction of the unexposed non-outcomes from the cohort. As we see in Table 7.9, the case-control OR is calculated as, $\dfrac{ad}{bc} = \dfrac{AgD}{gBC} = \dfrac{AD}{BC}$, which is exactly the cohort OR. Note that if we do *not* obtain all the cases, but instead a sample of f ($0 < f < 1$) of those cases (again without regard to exposure status), we would calculate the case-control OR as $\dfrac{ad}{bc} = \dfrac{fAgD}{gBfC} = \dfrac{AD}{BC}$, which is likewise unbiased.

Table 7.9 A CASE-CONTROL STUDY SAMPLED
FROM A COHORT STUDY SHOWN IN TABLE 7.8,
WITH CUMULATIVE SAMPLING OF CONTROLS

Case-control study	Cases	Controls	ccOR
Exposed	A	gB	$Ag D\,/\,gB\,C$
Not exposed	C	gD	

Table 7.10 A CASE-CONTROL STUDY SAMPLED FROM A COHORT STUDY
SHOWN IN TABLE 7.8, WITH CASE-COHORT CONTROL SAMPLING

Case-control study	Cases	Controls	ccOR
Exposed	A	$g(A + B)$	$A \, g(C + D) \, / \, g(A + B) \, C$
Not exposed	C	$g(C + D)$	

If the overall incidence of disease is low (usually, less than 10%, as in the commonly used heuristic called out in Chapter 2), then the cohort OR may provide a good estimate of the cohort RR; thus, under cumulative sampling and a rare disease assumption, the ccOR can estimate the (cohort OR which in turn estimates the) cohort RR. A common error is to assert that the rare disease assumption is *always necessary* for interpretation of the ccOR as the risk ratio, but that is not always the case, as our next sampling approach will demonstrate.

7.2.3.2 CASE-COHORT SAMPLING

In contrast, Table 7.6 demonstrates *case-cohort sampling*, in which we sample our controls from *among those who were at risk of the outcome at the beginning of follow-up*, again without regard for their true exposure status. When case-cohort sampling is used to select controls, the ccOR directly estimates the cohort risk ratio—regardless of the rare disease assumption.

Why should this be? Consider a second case-control study sampled from the cohort study in Table 7.8; we show this second case-control study in Table 7.10. As in cumulative sampling, we take all the cases, so $a = A$ and $c = C$ (Table 7.10). Then we turn to control sampling. Case-cohort sampling of controls considers only a sample (g) of the total people—cases and non-cases together—who were present at the baseline of the study. Since there were $A + B$ total exposed people at study baseline, our exposed controls $b = g(A + B)$; likewise $d = g(C + D)$. The case-control OR is calculated as, $\dfrac{ad}{bc} = \dfrac{Ag(C+D)}{g(A+B)C} = \dfrac{A(C+D)}{(A+B)C}$. This is less recognizable at first, but simple transformation reveals this quantity to be exactly $\dfrac{A/(A+B)}{C/(C+D)}$, which is the cohort risk ratio derived in Table 7.8.

Under case-cohort sampling, the ccOR estimates the cohort risk ratio even in absence of the rare disease assumption. To gain further intuition as to why, consider an additional numerical example in Table 7.11, in which the risk in the

Table 7.11 A COHORT STUDY (LEFT) AND A CASE-CONTROL STUDY UNDER CASE-COHORT SAMPLING (RIGHT)

Cohort study	Outcome		Total	Case-control study	Cases	Controls
	Yes	No				
Exposed	500	500	1,000	Exposed	500	125
Not exposed	250	750	1,000	Not exposed	250	125
Total	750	1,250	2,000			1,000

exposed is 50% and in the unexposed is 25%; the risk ratio is 2 (left panel). The cohort OR is $((500 \times 750) / (250 \times 500)) = 3$: quite different from the risk ratio because baseline risks of the outcome are quite high ($>>10\%$). Now suppose we enroll 1,000 people into a case-control study (right panel). First as cases, we enroll all 750 participants who experienced the outcome. Then we enroll 250 controls, selected from the total participants at the start of follow-up: at the start of follow-up there were 1,000 exposed and 1,000 unexposed individuals. If controls were selected without regard for exposure status, we would expect our controls to have the same 50% exposure prevalence seen in the original data, divided among our 250 total controls (right panel).

Calculating a ccOR from the right-hand 2×2 table yields $\dfrac{ad}{bc} = \dfrac{500 \times 125}{125 \times 250} = 2.00$, or exactly the same risk ratio as calculated on the left side *despite the lack of the rare-disease assumption*. The reader can now refer to the symbolic derivation of this result in Table 7.10.

One aspect of case-cohort sampling worth elucidating emerges from two premises. First, in this sampling approach, we sample controls from all cohort participants at baseline. Second, everyone who becomes a case (has the outcome) was a cohort participant at baseline. Therefore, under case-cohort sampling, it is possible for a single individual to appear in *both* the case *and* control groups; that is, in two cells of the case-control table. This may strike many readers as counterintuitive. But consider that the same thing is true of a risk—everyone in the numerator of a risk (who had the outcome in some time period) is also in the denominator (the same person was at risk at the start of that time period). Indeed, the fact that individuals can be both cases and controls under case-cohort sampling is *exactly why* case-cohort sampling allows direct estimation of the risk ratio.

7.2.3.3 INCIDENCE DENSITY SAMPLING

A third control-sampling scheme follows individuals through time and samples controls from the non-cases at the time each case occurs. For example, if a participant experiences a heart attack 1 month into the study, then we would select controls from among those individuals who had not yet experienced a heart attack at that moment. When the next heart attack occurred among study participants (2 weeks later, say) we would select controls from among the individuals *still* at risk of a heart attack. And so on. When controls are selected in this way, a type of *incidence density sampling* called *risk set sampling*, the ccOR directly estimates a hazard ratio (a measure we do not explore in this text, but see Hernán, 2010, for discussion), which can (under certain conditions) be interpreted as an incidence rate ratio as well.

Consider again a cancer registry–based study for cases of cancer from 1990 to 2010 in North Carolina. In this study, use of incidence density sampling would mean that, if we included a case of cancer diagnosed on March 1, 2005, we would identify a control or several controls living in North Carolina on the same date (or perhaps in a narrow window) who had not yet been diagnosed with cancer. Identifying such individuals may often be easier than identifying controls from all those living in North Carolina in 1990 who might become cases (essentially what case-cohort sampling would require).

7.3 CAUSAL INFERENCE IN CASE-CONTROL STUDIES

7.3.1 Temporality

As with retrospective cohort designs, case-control studies often begin only after outcomes have been identified—although (per the preceding example) this is not necessary. This will, of course, pose a similar challenge to establishing temporality: When exactly did an exposure begin, or end? When exactly did the outcome develop—what date should we assign as the incidence date? Such challenges are made simpler in a case-cohort design but warrant careful consideration.

7.3.2 Exchangeability and Positivity

The ability to identify causal effects in case-control studies depends on numerous factors, but the easiest way to think through the issues is by analogy to observational cohort studies. Like an observational cohort study, exposure is not randomized in a case-control study and so confounding is a threat to study validity. In Tables 7.1–7.11 above we have eschewed discussion of confounding to clarify the issues of control sampling and estimation, but confounding would be a threat to any of those case-control analyses exactly as it would be if we were analyzing the full cohort data.

Selection bias may likewise pose a threat to case-control studies and is generally recognized as a greater threat to case-control studies than to cohort studies. One particular concern is that while sampling of controls *should* be performed without regard to exposure status, this is not always the case. Biased sampling of the controls, such as sampling more exposed controls than unexposed controls, can easily lead to bias. We discuss one aspect of selection bias later, in Section 7.3.4 on causal diagrams for case-control studies and an additional problem that can arise when controls are sampled from clinics or hospitals in the Section 7.4.

As in a cohort study, if we must control for confounders, positivity may become an issue. However, there is no obvious reason why positivity should pose a greater threat in a case-control study setting than in a cohort study, except possibly that case-control studies are often smaller than cohort studies by design and so may, in practice, have more problems with empty cells (e.g., chance nonpositivity) than cohort studies.

7.3.3 Consistency

As in an observational cohort study, multiple versions of exposure (or treatment variation) may be an issue in a case-control study: without the strict control over treatment assignment which is given by design in a randomized trial, there may be substantial and important variation in exposures. Assessing variation in exposure may be more challenging in a case-control study than in a prospective observational cohort study if case-control exposures are assessed retrospectively. For example, it is difficult in a prospective setting to accurately ascertain how often someone takes nonsteroidal anti-inflammatory drugs (NSAIDs); it is

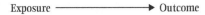

Exposure ──────────────▶ Outcome

Figure 7.1 Simplified directed acyclic graph for a cohort study.

straightforward to imagine how it would be more difficult to assess the same exposure which took place several years previously.

This is a time where the tradeoffs between measurement error and treatment variation may be more evident than at other times. Suppose we are studying the impact of use of NSAIDs on a pregnancy outcome and conduct the study among new mothers. If the exposure was "ever took more than 2 grams of NSAIDs on a single day during first trimester of pregnancy," it is easy to imagine substantial error being introduced in measurement back 9–12 months. We could eliminate much of that error by redefining exposure as "ever took any NSAIDs during first trimester of pregnancy"—it is more likely that people can remember ever-taking instead of number of ever-taking and what dose they took—but if there is strong dose–response effect on the outcome of interest, then such an exposure would hide important variation in treatment. Thus, in case-control studies with retrospective exposure measurement, it is critical to carefully define our exposures in terms of what we can reasonably measure.

7.3.4 Causal Diagrams for Case-Control Studies

The main factor differentiating a case-control study from a cohort study is sampling based on outcome status: regardless of control-sampling approach, we do not study all participants in the underlying population. Thus, while a cohort study causal diagram (omitting all other variables, including confounders of the exposure–disease relationship) might look like Figure 7.1, the case-control version of the same study would add a sampling (or selection) node (Figure 7.2). The arrow descending from the outcome into selection indicates that we sample into the study based on outcome status (e.g., all those with outcome = 1; not all those with outcome = 0).

It is illustrative to understand how this simple directed acyclic graph (DAG) maps to a 2 × 2 table for the same study: which is exactly what we show in Table 7.9. We recapitulate aspects of Table 7.9 as Table 7.12. When outcome affects sampling into the study, we expect to see only a proportion of those who did not experience the outcome (under cumulative sampling as in Table 7.12) or only a proportion of those present at baseline (under case-cohort sampling as shown in Table 7.10, and not recapitulated in Table 7.12).

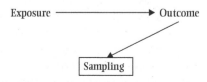

Exposure ──────────────▶ Outcome
                                              ╱
                              ┌──────────┐◀╱
                              │ Sampling │
                              └──────────┘

Figure 7.2 Simplified directed acyclic graph for a case-control study.

Table 7.12 CUMULATIVE SAMPLING FROM A COHORT STUDY (LEFT) TO
A CASE-CONTROL STUDY (RIGHT) ENSURES THAT THE CASE-CONTROL
ODDS RATIO () ESTIMATES THE COHORT ODDS RATIO

Cohort study	Outcome		Total	Case-control study	Cases	Controls	
	Yes	No					
Exposed	A	B	$A + B$	Exposed	A	gB	$A + gB$
Not exposed	C	D	$C + D$	Not exposed	C	gD	$C + gD$
Risk difference	$\dfrac{A}{A+B} - \dfrac{C}{C+D}$			Risk difference (biased)	$\dfrac{A}{A+gB} - \dfrac{C}{C+gD}$		
Risk ratio	$(\dfrac{A}{A+B}) / (\dfrac{C}{C+D})$			Risk ratio (biased)	$(\dfrac{A}{A+gB}) / (\dfrac{C}{C+gD})$		
Odds ratio	$\dfrac{AD}{CB}$			Odds ratio (unbiased)	$\dfrac{AgD}{CgB}$		

We can calculate the risk difference and risk ratio from Table 7.12 as well as the OR: for example, the risk difference is $\dfrac{A}{A+gB} - \dfrac{C}{C+gD}$ and the risk ratio is $\dfrac{A}{A+gB} / \dfrac{C}{C+gD}$. Except in special cases such as when $g = 1$ (at which point we are no longer sampling controls and so are simply performing a cohort study), neither the risk difference nor risk ratio estimated from the case control study (right) will estimate the cohort risk difference or risk ratio (left).

In truth, this is what we should expect: Wacholder referred to the case-control study as giving us a kind of "data missing by design," in that, by design we sample only a fraction of the non-cases (or combined cases and non-cases) in the parent cohort study, and the remainder are missing (Wacholder, 1996).[1] Indeed, compare Figure 7.2 to Figure 3.6 (right panel): while the context is different, the causal structure is the same, in which inclusion in our analysis is conditional on outcome status. So it is not surprising that the risk difference and risk ratio are biased in a case-control study with cumulative sampling (Table 7.12). What *is* surprising is that the case-control OR is an *unbiased* estimate of the cohort OR. There are numerous ways to understand why the OR is not biased in Table 7.12; perhaps the simplest is that the mathematical structure of the OR allows the sampling fractions (g) to cancel.

---

[1] Recent/ongoing work in using causal diagrams for missing data suggest that it might be more accurate to think of this as "data missing by design under complete case analysis," and likewise that it may be important to consider issues of effect measure modification of the case-control odds ratio closely in analysis.

7.4 REAL CASE-CONTROL STUDIES

For the most part we have been describing ideal case-control studies in which a case-control study is nested inside an established, prospective observational cohort study. This, however, is a best-case scenario. When a case-control study is nested within an established cohort, the cohort population is well-defined and fully characterized. The cases are fully enumerated, and information about the participants has usually been captured in real-time, which precludes the need to ask participants to recall long-ago exposures. When a case-control study is conducted outside of an established cohort, it may present substantially more challenges.

7.4.1 Identification of Controls

In more realistic settings, it is often easier to begin by identifying cases—from a cancer registry, or a hospital, or the community. Just as often, it is more difficult in such settings to identify controls.

   In practice, one common approach is to identify cases from a hospital or clinic setting and then to subsequently sample controls from the same setting. For example, cases might be those admitted to a hospital after a heart attack, while controls might be sampled from among those at the same hospital who were admitted for another reason. In the United States, this is often cited as an approach to help match on access to healthcare; it is certainly a *convenient* way to proceed. However, the flaws with this approach were pointed out initially in 1946, by Berkson. Briefly, this approach is problematic in that individuals who are in a hospital do not typically represent the population from which the cases arose: for example, controls selected from the hospital are likely to have more access to healthcare than individuals in the general population and likewise more "health-seeking behavior." We can also view this so-called *Berkson's bias* through the lens of collider bias (Snoep, Morabia, Hernández-Díaz, Hernán, & Vandenbroucke, 2014), and broadly this issue is considered by many to be a form of selection bias (Hernán, Hernández-Díaz, & Robins, 2004).

   More useful in identifying controls, generally, is to consider the imaginary or theoretical cohort in which the case-control study is nested and then ask whether the controls represent that cohort study appropriately. Depending on the specific research question, it may be more or less straightforward to imagine what the analogous cohort study would have looked like and thus which controls truly represent the population from which the cases arose.

7.4.2 Limitations of Case-Control Studies

Many of the potential limitations of observational cohort studies also apply to case-control studies—and are sometimes amplified due to the retrospective nature of data collection that often occurs with case-control designs. Here, we expand briefly on limitations specific to case-control designs compared with observational cohort designs.

When case-control studies are conducted backward in time (which is most often how they are conducted)—first identifying existing cases and only then figuring out long-ago exposure conditions—the potential for exposure misclassification is almost certainly higher than in a prospective setting. Not only might the outcome status of individuals be known (and thus introduce bias into the outcome assessment) but asking participants to recall long-ago exposures is fraught with the possibility of flawed recall. Such problems with recall may have to do with simple lapses in memory, but recall bias may also arise differentially based on outcome status. One example is in case-control studies of birth defects, in which mothers of infants with a congenital abnormality are thought to over-recall drug exposures (because, it is speculated, they are looking for a reason to explain the abnormality; see Rockenbauer et al., 2001, for a report).

Related, if cases are identified based on outcome status, then, of course, blinded assessment of the outcome may not be possible: the exception to this is if outcomes have been collected for reasons outside the study (as in a death registry or cancer registry), and so in effect outcome assessment was blinded to study hypothesis. As well, retrospective assessment of exposure may make exposure more difficult to assess with blinding; if exposure status is evaluated by individuals unaware of outcome status (and not by the study investigators) blinding may remain possible.

7.4.3 Advantages of Case-Control Studies

With these limitations come specific advantages. As we noted earlier, case-control studies can be extremely efficient in the context of constrained resources. In particular, case-control studies may be efficient in the number of people we need to enroll (which would be of concern if exposure ascertainment was costly), but also in the length of time we have to wait before we can get an answer to a pressing public health question (because we can begin the study after outcomes have occurred and been collected).

The fact that we can always think of case-control studies as nested within a cohort study (even if that cohort study is implicit) suggests that the routine placement of case-control studies under cohort studies on hierarchies of study designs is not well-founded. Indeed, there are numerous shared issues between these two study designs with respect to challenges in causal inference (e.g., confounding remains a similar issue between the two). And case-control designs can bring enormously increased efficiency. Thus, overall, case-control studies should not, broadly and universally, be considered inferior designs.

7.5 ANALYSIS OF CASE-CONTROL STUDIES

As we discussed in Section 7.1, our main goal in case-control studies is to estimate the case-control OR. Here, we briefly discuss two calculations related to the OR.

First we explain how to calculate the 95% confidence limit for the OR. Then, we explain the Mantel-Haenszel calculation for the OR to adjust for confounding.

7.5.1 Calculation of 95% CIs of the ORs

This book does not dwell deeply on the issue of variance, but for case-control studies (as noted earlier) introducing a basic variance calculation will be helpful. The critical thing you need to understand for this calculation is the natural log function (ln), which is a log function in base e ($\log_e$, rather than the more typical $\log_{10}$). e, you may recall, is an irrational number approximately equal to 2.71828, and it pops up regularly in the sciences (most beautifully in Euler's equation, $e^{i\pi} + 1 = 0$); $\ln(x)$ asks the question: To what power do we raise e, in order to obtain x?

Knowing this, you will now be able to interpret the formula for the variance of the natural log of OR, which is

$$Var(\ln(OR)) = \frac{1}{a} + \frac{1}{b} + \frac{1}{c} + \frac{1}{d}$$

and so the standard error (SE) of the natural log of the OR is the square root of the variance, or

$$SE(\ln(OR)) = \sqrt{\frac{1}{a} + \frac{1}{b} + \frac{1}{c} + \frac{1}{d}}$$

The variance and SE can be calculated from the data in Table 7.1 as

$$Var(\ln(OR)) = \frac{1}{200} + \frac{1}{1800} + \frac{1}{100} + \frac{1}{1900} = 0.0161,$$

and so

$$SE(\ln(OR)) = \sqrt{\frac{1}{200} + \frac{1}{1800} + \frac{1}{100} + \frac{1}{1900}} = 0.1268.$$

We use that SE along with the OR itself to calculate a lower 95% confidence limit of the OR in the full data of Table 7.1 as follows:

$$LCL_{95} = \exp(\ln(OR) - 1.96(SE(\ln(OR))))$$

where

$$\ln(OR) = \ln(2.11111) = 0.7472$$

and therefore

$$LCL_{95} = \exp(0.7472 - 1.96(0.1268)) = 1.6465$$

The UCL is calculated similarly, as

$$UCL_{95} = \exp(\ln(OR) + 1.96(SE(\ln(OR))))$$

and therefore

$$UCL_{95} = \exp(0.7472 + 1.96(0.1268)) = 2.7068$$

Thus, for the OR of 2.11 calculated from Table 7.1, we would calculate 95% CIs of (1.65, 2.71). Similar calculations apply to data in subsequent tables.

7.5.2 Mantel-Haenzsel Estimator for ORs

As in the previous chapter, we can use Mantel-Haenzsel approaches to calculate a confounding-adjusted OR when we are willing to assume homogeneity (i.e., that the OR at one level of the confounder is essentially the same as on the other levels of the confounder). For a level of a covariate indicated by $Z = z$, the Mantel-Haenszel OR equation (Mantel & Haenszel, 1959; Rothman, Greenland, & Lash, 2008) is:

$$\widehat{OR}_{mh} = \frac{\sum_z \left\{ a_z d_z / n_i \right\}}{\sum_z \left\{ c_z b_z / n_i \right\}}, n_i = a_i + b_i + c_i + d_i$$

7.6 REVIEWING A CASE-CONTROL STUDY

While much of the approach to the review of a case-control study is similar to that of a cohort study(e.g., it is asking a specific and actionable public health question), there are a few points specific to case-control studies themselves.

1. A key idea in reviewing a case-control study is to ask, first, is this study nested inside an actual cohort? If so, what is that cohort, and why was a case-control approach used, instead of a cohort design? If not, can you identify an implicit or ideal cohort, inside of which the case-control study was nested? Either way, what is the cohort study that would have been performed here if it was possible?

2. How were controls sampled? Given this, what cohort effect estimate will be estimated by the case-control OR? Do the authors correctly identify this measure and/or correctly interpret the OR from their own study?

3. Do the authors acknowledge the potential limitations of a case-control design (e.g., the need to collect exposure and covariate data from

historical records or from interviews asking people to recall exposures in the past) without dipping into cynicism about the case-control design? Recall, case-control designs can be equally as valid as prospective observational cohort designs, even while being far more efficient.

7.7 SUMMARY

Case-control studies are the third of the three central study designs we consider in this textbook. Like both randomized trials and observational cohort studies, case-control studies have both advantages and disadvantages for assessing causal effects. On the positive side, they can be viewed as a highly efficient way of conducting a cohort study, efficient in both cost and time to complete (especially if studying outcomes which have already occurred). On the other hand, like cohort studies, case-control studies may suffer from uncontrolled confounding; as well, case-control studies conducted after the occurrence of outcome may be more prone to recall or measurement biases, especially of long-ago exposures or confounders.

These relative advantages and disadvantages of each study design are something to keep in mind as you read the next and final chapter in Section II of this book, in which we briefly consider several additional study designs.

REFERENCES

Berkson, J. (1946). Limitations of the application of fourfold table analysis to hospital data. *Biometrics Bulletin*, *2*(3), 47–53.

Hernán, M. A. (2010). The hazards of hazard ratios. *Epidemiology*, *21*(1), 13–15.

Hernán, M. A., Hernández-Díaz, S., & Robins, J. M. (2004). A structural approach to selection bias. *Epidemiology*, *15*(5), 615–625.

Lane-Claypon, J. E. (1926). A further report on cancer of the breast with special reference to its associated antecedent conditions. *London: Ministry of Health. Reports on Public Health and Medical Subjects.*, *32*, 189.

Mantel, N., & Haenszel, M. W. (1959). Statistical aspects of thee analysis of data from retrospective studies of disease. *Journal of the National Cancer Institute*, *22*, 719–748.

Paneth, N., Susser, E., & Susser, M. (2002a). Origins and early development of the case-control study: Part 1, Early evolution. *Soz Praventivmed*, *47*(5), 282–288.

Paneth, N., Susser, E., & Susser, M. (2002b). Origins and early development of the case-control study: Part 2, The case-control study from Lane-Claypon to 1950. *Soz Praventivmed*, *47*(6), 359–365.

Rockenbauer, M., Olsen, J., Czeizel, A. E., Pedersen, L., Sørensen, H. T.; EuroMAP Group. (2001). Recall bias in a case-control surveillance system on the use of medicine during pregnancy. *Epidemiology*, *12*(4), 461–466.

Rothman, K. J., Greenland, S., & Lash, T. L. (2008). *Modern epidemiology* (3rd ed.). Philadelphia: Lippincott Williams & Wilkins.

Snoep, J. D., Morabia, A., Hernández-Díaz, S., Hernán, M. A., & Vandenbroucke, J. P. (2014). Commentary: A structural approach to Berkson's fallacy and a guide to a history of opinions about it. *International Journal of Epidemiology*, *43*(2), 515–521. doi:10.1093/ije/dyu026

Wacholder, S. (1996). The case-control study as data missing by design: Estimating risk differences. *Epidemiology*, *7*(2), 144–150.

8

Other Study Designs

In this brief chapter, we describe several additional study designs beyond those covered at more length in previous chapters. None of the explanations in this chapter is complete. Our goal, rather, is to give you a passing knowledge of general concepts and a basis for deciding whether such designs may be worth more study later.

We first describe some more "traditional" epidemiologic designs, among them case reports and series, case-crossover studies, and cross-sectional studies. Next, we describe several "hybrid" designs that combine aspects of randomized trials with aspects of observational studies—including systematic reviews and meta-analyses, which are observational studies of study results—often including randomized trial results. Finally, we introduce the idea of *quasi-experiments*, which are themselves a sort of hybrid in which observational data yields conditions close to what we might see in a randomized experiment.

8.1 TRADITIONAL DESIGNS

8.1.1 Case Reports and Case Series

A case report (or case study) is simply a description, often narrative, of a particular case—usually of disease. A case series is similar but involves several such narratives, usually with some key commonality that makes them of interest, particularly to clinicians. There is a long history of such reports: case reports have been found in Egyptian papyrus dating to approximately 1600 BCE as well as in the writings of Hippocrates, circa 400 BCE (Nissen & Wynn, 2014).

Case reports usually wind up at the bottom of hierarchies of study designs, if they are listed at all—but such placement overlooks the fact that such studies are extremely good at certain sorts of causal inference. In particular, a case report (recounted accurately, we note!) is all that is necessary to prove that something is not always true, in the way that the single observation of a black swan can prove that not all swans are white. Case reports and case studies can also alert public health researchers and the public generally of emerging infectious diseases, as with the initial case report of five young men in 1981, all of whom suffered from a disease (*Pneumocystis carinii* pneumonia) more typical of people

Epidemiology by Design: A Causal Approach to the Health Sciences. Daniel Westreich, Oxford University Press (2020). © Oxford University Press.
DOI: 10.1093/oso/9780190665760.001.0001

receiving long-term immunosuppressive therapy than otherwise healthy young men (Centers for Disease Control [CDC], 1981). This was, of course, the first report of the AIDS epidemic in the medical literature.

The danger of case studies and case series is that the human mind is prone to overvaluing narrative and anecdotal evidence and relatively undervaluing statistical evidence; as such, we often attach great significance to stories. Much public suspicion about a link between vaccines and autism can be traced back to the (now-withdrawn) case series published in *The Lancet* (which we deliberately do not cite here); although reporting by the *British Medical Journal* credibly accuses the lead author of that article of scientific fraud (Deer, 2011; Godlee, Smith, & Marcovitch, 2011), nonetheless the perception that there is a link persists—in part because of the power of a good story.

8.1.2 Case-Crossover

A case-crossover study is an innovative design first published by Maclure (1991) and appropriate to very short-term exposures—often exposures whose effects "wash out" quickly. This design allows individuals to serve as their own controls by comparing exposed and unexposed person-time. The classic example was Mittelman et al.'s (1993) application to elucidate how heavy physical exertion was an immediate trigger of myocardial infarction (MI). These authors interviewed patients who had suffered an MI about their activity in the 26 hours prior to heart attack and compared the physical activity in those periods (did the participant have heavy activity or light?) with physical activity in other time periods after which an MI did not occur.

This design is in some ways an observational analogue of the crossover randomized trial. In a classic such trial, which would be optimal for a short-term exposure and transient outcome, individuals might be randomized to one of two active treatments (A or B) for a short period (weeks or months), stopped on their treatment, and then (after a reset or washout period), started on the other active treatment (B or A) (Maclure & Mittleman, 2000).

The applications for the case-crossover design are somewhat limited, but the tool is extremely useful when appropriate (Maclure, 2007). For example, we could use the design to study the effects of texting while driving on risk of car accident or of smoking, alcohol, or drug-use on a short-term outcome such as heart attack or stroke.

8.1.3 Cross-Sectional Study

A cross-sectional study is essentially one in which all measurements are performed at the same time—or at least over a small window in time. As such, cross-sectional studies are appropriate for assessing associations but are not generally useful in assessing causality. The exception is when data can be captured cross-sectionally such that the exposure and outcome have a clear time ordering, as would be the case with an exposure during infancy (supposing that participants can recall the exposure in question) and an outcome of present-day blood pressure among adults. Thus, cross-sectional studies are most useful for assessing associations (as in Chapter 2) as well as in descriptive and predictive epidemiology more broadly (Chapter 4), although all of these can also be pursued in longitudinal cohorts as well.

8.2 HYBRID DESIGNS

Hybrid designs are those that include both randomized and observational components. Here, we review several such designs to give the reader a sense of what is possible. We include systematic reviews and meta-analysis in this section, even though these are studies of previously conducted studies rather than of individuals. However, these designs are critically important to understanding epidemiologic evidence. They are appropriate for this section because while such studies may limit their scope to previously published randomized studies, both begin by observing what studies have been published in the literature.

8.2.1 Pragmatic Trials

A pragmatic trial is, essentially, a randomized trial which is already scaled up and implemented—as close as possible to what might be implemented in other settings down the road. For example, while a typical individually randomized clinical trial will have strict inclusion and exclusion criteria, a pragmatic trial will typically try to include exactly those individuals to whom the intervention is meant to apply after it is scaled up. The pragmatic trial would not, for example, exclude individuals with substantial comorbidities, nor enrich trial enrollment for those at highest risk of the outcome. Thus, while still randomized, pragmatic trials often look more like observational studies in many ways.

Pragmatic trials are typically much larger than traditional trials and (hand-in-hand with this fact) typically test a version of the intervention which works at this larger scale—and thus, if it works in the pragmatic trial, can be scaled up to the whole target population immediately, with few (if any) changes. For example, an individually randomized trial of pre-exposure prophylaxis for HIV using antiretroviral therapy might involve intensive initial and follow-up counseling about the use of the medication for each individual participant. Such individual counseling may be difficult to scale up to cover the whole population of a country; thus, a more pragmatic version of that intervention might rely on group counseling sessions. The pragmatic trial, then, might use group counseling.

As will become more evident in Chapter 9, pragmatic trials, nested in the target population, including study populations which are highly representative of that target, and using a version of the intervention which is likely extremely similar to what could be scaled up, are highly relevant to bridging the gap between the effect of an exposure in a study sample and the effect of an intervention against that exposure in a target population.

8.2.2 Doubly Randomized Preference Trials

Doubly randomized preference trials (DRPTs) are a useful method when we wish to study both the causal effects of assignment of an intervention and also the effects of *choice* of that same intervention—and whether the effect of an intervention might differ based on whether it is assigned compared to whether it is chosen.

Consider that we wish to obtain evidence about the impact of diet on weight loss, comparing a low-fat and a low-carbohydrate diet. The DRPT design proceeds by, first, randomizing participants into two arms: a "choice" arm, in which participants are educated about both arms of the trial and invited to choose the diet they think will work best for them, and a "second randomization" arm, in which participants are randomized into either a low-fat or low-carb diet. All individuals are followed-up. The *first* randomization yields exchangeability (in expectation) between participants allowed to choose their diet and participants who were randomized to a specific diet. The *second* randomization further guarantees exchangeability between those participants who were randomized to a low-fat diet and participants randomized to a low-carb diet.

In addition, however, we can compare the effect of a low-carb diet among those randomized to that diet to the effect of that diet among those who chose that diet. Differences between those can be partly ascribed to confounding or treatment variation. For example, if a low-carb diet works better among those who choose that diet, it might be because, in choosing that diet, people tend to adhere to the diet better than if they are assigned to it.

Aspects of the DRPT as well as pragmatic trials can be integrated into more traditional randomized trials. Suppose an investigator wants to run a trial to see if self-testing for some disease is a viable approach. One trial that we could run would randomize patients either to standard of care (testing in clinic) verus self-testing: effectively asking, what if we didn't change the standard of care at all, compared to what if we shifted to exclusive self-testing? But unless we are considering abandoning clinic-testing in favor of exclusive self-testing, this comparison may not give us the information we want. A more likely policy outcome would be to give patients the option of self-testing; thus, a better trial might be randomization to standard of care compared with randomization to the participant's choice of standard of care or self-testing. This comparison maps very closely to the policy that might be subsequently implemented and also allows us to investigate the process of choosing one option over another.

8.2.3 Systematic Review

A systematic review of the literature is a study of other studies—an organized search of the (usually peer-reviewed) literature to see what has been written about a particular subject. Ideally, systematic reviews are conducted by establishing literature search parameters (e.g., key phrases) and a standardized approach to evaluating the results of the search. Often systematic reviews are limited a priori to published randomized trials or published literature generally; sometimes they include the so-called gray literature, which includes unpublished works such as conference abstracts and white papers. A related, key difficulty in conducting a systematic review arises when reviewers start to consider the quality of papers to include in the review, for example rejecting observational studies which do not control for key confounders. Judging paper quality is, of course, subjective: transparency in reporting and applying any quality criteria is key to the validity of the resulting review (Reeves, Koppel, Barr, Freeth, & Hammick, 2002).

Systematic reviews are an excellent way to understand the state of the science on a specific topic; they may or may not lead directly to meta-analysis. The Preferred Reporting Items for Systematic Reviews and Meta-Analyses (PRISMA) statement gives additional information about how to conduct a systematic review, as well as how to conduct a meta-analysis (Moher, Liberati, Tetzlaff, Altman, & Group, 2009).

8.2.4 Meta-Analysis

A meta-analysis, like a systematic review, is a study of other, previously conducted studies (Grant & Booth, 2009). Typically, the meta-analysis is the study of the *results* of those studies rather than the *data* from those studies. Generally, the purpose of a meta-analysis is to harness the "wisdom of crowds" by combining results from multiple studies (generally, resulting from a systematic review) into a single estimate. As with many subjects touched on briefly in this text, numerous papers and indeed entire other textbooks have been written on meta-analysis; here, we only very briefly discuss the methodological pitfalls of meta-analysis as it is frequently conducted in the literature.

Broadly, a meta-analysis proceeds as follows (a full checklist is available as part of PRISMA; Moher et al., 2009): the investigator selects a question, often one about the magnitude of a specific exposure–outcome relationship (e.g., What is the risk ratio for all-cause mortality comparing individuals taking a daily statin to those not taking a statin?). A systematic review is then conducted of the literature (see earlier discussion) to identify relevant studies for inclusion. Then the essential information is abstracted from each study. Such information includes, most centrally, the estimated effect of the exposure on the outcome from the study, but often includes other information as well, such as study size and details of how the study was conducted.

At this point, the investigator will frequently evaluate the heterogeneity of effect estimates; if the results are quite heterogeneous, the investigator may reject the idea of performing a meta-analysis altogether because combining heterogeneous study results may be misleading to readers (Scott, Greenberg, Poole, & Campbell, 2006). If the investigator wishes to proceed, however, she can then combine the estimates of effect (e.g., the risk differences, risk ratios, or hazard ratios) abstracted from the studies using a statistical technique such as inverse-variance weighting (Rothman, Greenland, & Lash, 2008). Sometimes investigators will account for variability in study results by examining patterns in that variability by study characteristics, such as variations in exposure definitions, setting, study design, or participant characteristics, a process which often involves *meta-regression* (Rothman et al., 2008).

Earlier, we noted that meta-analyses (and systematic reviews) start from observing the already-published literature, even if the meta-analysis is concentrating on randomized trials. But studies are conducted—and published— in ways which may lead to certain types of studies not being published at higher rates. For example, historically, it has been difficult to publish "null findings"; that is, the risk differences (or ratios) statistically indistinguishable from the null value of 0 (or 1). Thus, the results of a meta-analysis may be biased due to a form of study selection bias usually termed *publication bias*. Statistical techniques exist to help diagnose and possibly correct for the presence of publication bias although certain approaches to meta-analysis can amplify such biases as well (Greenland, 1994; Rothman et al., 2008).

One variation on meta-analysis is sometimes called an *individual patient data meta-analysis*, in which, rather than analyzing the risk ratios from each of N studies, the investigator obtains the original data from all N studies, pools that data, and reanalyzes the individual data. Such analyses usually allow for clustering of effects by original study and have some advantages over traditional meta-analysis: for example, in observational settings, the investigator can condition on a common set of variables across all studies.

8.3 QUASI-EXPERIMENTS

Quasi-experimental designs are a large and important class of approaches to estimation of causal effects that historically—and only broadly speaking—have been more popular in economics, public policy, and political science contexts than they have been in epidemiology and public health (Barnighausen et al., 2017; Bor, 2016).

Quasi-experiments are approaches to effect estimation in which investigators identify (or create) a source of variation in the exposure which is unrelated to the rest of the causal system under study—including the outcome (except through the exposure itself) and the confounders. One such source of variation is external policies such as laws, especially in such cases when laws are passed in comparable locations such as neighboring counties at different times. Another is arbitrary cutoffs on linear scales: nothing magical happens to a young adult's brain between the ages of 20 years 11 months and 21 years—but in the United States, that 1 month leads to a vastly increased access to alcohol due to existing laws. Still another is random natural variation (as in genetics) or randomly occurring events beyond the control of the individuals affected (such as experiencing a bus accident). Such sources of variation create what are often called *quasi-* or sometimes *natural experiments* (Bor, 2016).

In the remainder of this section and chapter, we discuss several specific designs, but first we provide some history on these methods.

8.3.1 Natural Experiments: An Origin Story

This is where we finally discuss Dr. John Snow (1813–1858). Snow was a physician in London in the mid-19th century, famous early on for his work in introducing anesthesia to general clinical practice: indeed, he administered chloroform to Queen Victoria in 1853 during childbirth (Ramsay, 2006). Snow, through previous epidemics of cholera in London, had formulated the (correct) hypothesis that cholera was transmitted not through air (as was widely supposed) but through water. As this was an era in which human waste was routinely flushed into the same Thames River from which water supplies were often drawn, Snow further hypothesized that the Thames around London was a key component in the epidemic (Bynum, 2013; Johnson, 2006).

To Snow's eternal credit, he recognized two key facts. First, that there were two water companies serving an area of London near the Broad Street Pump: the Southwark and Vauxhall Company, which drew from the dirty river of central London, and the Lambeth Company, which drew from the upriver, cleaner section of the Thames. And, second, that there were no patterns among individuals who got their water from one company or another and no relation between which company you received your water from, and who you were: that is, whether you were rich or poor, young or old, working or not. As Snow put this second point,

> In the sub-districts enumerated in the above table as being supplied by both Companies, the mixing of the supply is of the most intimate kind. The pipes of each Company go down all the streets, and into nearly all the courts and alleys. A few houses are supplied by one Company and a few by the other, according to the decision of the owner or occupier at that time when the Water Companies were in active competition. In many cases a single house has a supply different from that on either side. Each company supplies both rich and poor, both large houses and small; there is no difference either in the condition or occupation of the persons receiving the water of the different Companies. (Snow, 1855)

In modern terms, of course, this second point relates to confounding: Snow was arguing that who supplied your water was not confounded by wealth, by house size, or by the "condition or occupation of the persons" receiving the water.

Snow then observed much higher risks of cholera (and death) among those served by the Southwark and Vauxhall than those served by Lambeth, and since—as he argued—there was no confounding of the water exposure–cholera relationship, he interpreted this natural experiment as a causal effect. Policy—his

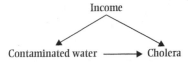

Figure 8.1 A directed acyclic graph for a simple study of the effect of contaminated water on cholera infection.

recommendation to the water board to remove the pump handle—followed (and soon after officials put it right back: the frustration of the epidemiologist in trying to influence policy also has its origins in this story). For more reading on Snow, Ramsay et al. (2006) provides an overview, and Steven Berlin Johnson's book *The Ghost Map* provides a "tick-tock" of the events (Johnson, 2006).[1]

8.3.2 Instrumental Variables

Instrumental variables are probably the best known and most widely used quasi-experimental method within epidemiology and are in fact easily understood through the lens of Snow's story. Consider that Snow's hypothesis was "exposure to contaminated water is the cause of cholera," a hypothesis that could be shown as a directed acyclic graph (DAG), as in Figure 8.1, with possible confounding by Income: perhaps Income affects the probability of being exposed to Contaminated water (if uncontaminated water, piped over a longer distance, were more expensive and in consequence only purchased by wealthier people), and perhaps Income also somehow affects your risk of Cholera (if rich people could afford to drink more alcohol, likewise reducing risks of infection).

Of course, this is not the study Snow did: he did the study shown in Figure 8.2. In this DAG, whether or not you were exposed to Contaminated water may still be caused by Income, but (i) exposure is (also) caused by which Company gave you your water (and, in the subdistricts Snow studied, it might be argued that in fact the arrow from Income to Contaminated water was entirely absent: that the only cause of exposure to Contaminated water was Company). In addition, the DAG reflects that (ii) which of the Companies gave you your water is unrelated to Income—as well as other characteristics that might confound the relationship between exposure to Contaminated water and Cholera.

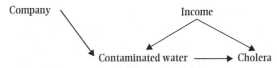

Figure 8.2 Adding to Figure 8.1 that Company affects contaminated water exposure.

1. Also consider visiting the John Snow Pub if you happen to be in London.

Had Snow wanted to study the effect of contaminated water per se, then he would have had to contend with confounding. As it was, he was studying the effect of Company—which, regardless of whether Income affects exposure in Snow's setting, is clearly a very good proxy for exposure—on Cholera outcomes. We see from Figure 8.2 that there is no confounding of the Company → Cholera causal relationship: there are no unblocked back door paths between them.

What Snow did was not quite an instrumental variable analysis, but it was close: had Snow used the effect of Company on Cholera as a means of estimating the effect of Contaminated water (not which company, but the contaminated water itself) on Cholera, then it might have been. To do such an analysis, Snow would have had to meet several general conditions for an instrument variable analysis: namely, that (a) the instrument has a causal effect on the exposure, that (b) there is no confounding of the instrument and the outcome, and (c) that the effect of the instrument on the outcome is entirely through the exposure (Hernán & Robins, 2006). As is immediately clear, point (i) above meets general condition (a) and point (ii) above meets general condition (b). If we believe Figure 8.2, that the only way that the company which delivers your water affects your cholera risk is via the water it delivers to you, the we meet condition (c) as well, and we can consider Company an instrumental variable.

Another way to think about instrumental variable analysis is in terms of a randomized trial. Suppose we want to understand the impact of use of statins on risk of heart attack, but we are concerned about confounding by age of those taking statins. One solution to this is to randomize who is assigned to take statins and who is not: since assignment to statin is randomized, it can be expected to be structurally independent of Age (hence no arrow from Age to Randomized assignment in Figure 8.3). You may note that Randomized assignment meets general conditions (a), (b), and (c) and may thus be considered an instrumental variable—randomized treatment assignment, then, can be thought of as an artificially created instrumental variable.

From our randomized trial discussion (Chapter 5), we recall that we can conduct an intention-to-treat (ITT) analysis, examining the effect of assignment to statin on risk of stroke without considering confounding by age, or we can conduct a compliance-corrected analysis, examining the effect of actual statin use on risk of stroke, but we must consider confounding by age. Here, we propose that we can use randomized statin assignment as an instrumental variable to assess (under additional assumptions, see earlier discussion and Hernán and Robins,

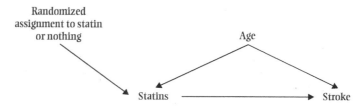

Figure 8.3 A directed acyclic graph for a randomized trial of statins on stroke risk.

2006) the effect of actual statin use on risk of stroke *without* explicitly accounting for age.

It is important to remember that most randomized trials simply perform an ITT analysis, which estimates the effect of treatment assignment and does not treat the randomized assignment as an instrumental variable per se: in a typical instrumental variable analysis we are usually interested not in the effect of the instrument per se, but rather in using the instrument only to get information about the effect of the underlying exposure. As such, the target of a typical instrumental variable analysis generally falls closer to what is estimated in compliance-corrected analysis rather than in ITT analysis. However, the instrumental variable analysis does not exactly estimate the former: rather, it typically estimates a complier-average causal effect, which is (broadly) the effect among those who, when they receive assignment to statin, take statin. Note that the *complier average causal effect* is similar, but not identical to, what many people typically mean by a "per-protocol" effect in a randomized trial setting.

When they can be identified, then, instrumental variables may be an "epidemiologist's dream" (Hernán & Robins, 2006), although using poor or imperfect instruments while believing they are good instrumental variables can lead to bias. A critical error sometimes made with instrumental variables is believing incorrectly that there is no other pathway between the instrument and the outcome in addition to the exposure of interest: when this is violated, use of an instrumental variable can lead to significant bias.

8.3.3 Difference in Differences

The difference in difference method is an approach to estimating the impact of an external policy (frequently, a law) passed in one setting but not another by looking at trends in some outcome variable before and after the passage of the policy in a group affected by the policy and a control group which is not expected to be affected (Bärnighausen et al., 2017).

For example, if a policy mandating bicycle helmets is passed in one county but not in a neighboring county, then we could examine trends over time of bicycle injuries in both counties—before and after the law passed. In a broad sense, if the rate of injury falls in the affected county after the law passes but not in the unaffected county, we might attribute the fall to the law. But what if the rate of injury falls in both counties? Then we can ask: Did rates fall under the law more than we would have expected them to fall without the law, given how much rates fell in the control county? Of course, in reality, we would be very hesitant to make strong conclusions based only on a single county!

The difference in differences approach to inference is not, from appearances, an instrumental variable approach, in that interest remains in the effect of the policy per se, not in the effect of the policy on some exposure (e.g., on the law mandating bicycle helmets—not on how many bicycle helmets were worn in the county). Instead, we might think of the difference in difference method as a "found" randomized trial: we begin with a single, active arm of a randomized trial—we have a county, and we passed a law—and then we search for an appropriate control arm for that active arm. Broadly, the key assumptions of identifying that control group is that other factors influencing the outcome (injuries, say) are similar in both counties and that differences between the counties are not changing over time (Bärnighausen et al., 2017).

8.3.4 Regression Discontinuity

Regression discontinuity leverages the arbitrariness of certain clinical thresholds. When treatments function cutoff values—for example, "if hemoglobin falls below 11 g/dL, treat with iron supplementation" or "if CD4 count falls below 200 cells/mm³ in a patient with HIV, initiate antiretroviral therapy"—then we can observe quite different outcomes for certain conditions on either side of that cutoff. The definition of poverty is similarly an arbitrary cutoff on a linear scale of income, but which side of that cutoff one falls on may give one access to certain economic or social benefits (such as food stamps) and thus could be used to test the impact of those benefits.

Consider two people, M and K: M has a true hemoglobin of 10.9 g/dL, while K has a true hemoglobin of 11.1 g/dL. These two people have very similar health statuses—the 0.2 g/dL difference in hemoglobin has little to no impact on health, and natural variation within a day may be as much as 10 times that amount. But one of these individuals will be given iron supplementation and the other will not. Thus, all other things being equal (e.g., individuals of the same sex, age, health status otherwise), we could see this as a two-person randomized trial. After all, if we believe that the difference between the hemoglobin levels of the two individuals is immaterial, then we might consider the assignment of treatment among those two individuals to be *as good as random*. This argument can go even further if the measurement error in an assay is greater than the variation in the study.

The great disadvantage of regression discontinuity models is that they only identify causal effects among those right at the discontinuity threshold: in this case, the regression discontinuity approach might only identify the causal effect of iron supplementation among those with a hemoglobin of exactly 11 g/dL (or exactly, plus or minus measurement error)—a more limited conclusion than one might prefer. While careful assumptions may allow the analyst to make inferences about—for example—the effect of iron supplementation on those with a hemoglobin of 10.5, 10.0, or 8.2 g/dL, such extrapolations must be done quite carefully. Understanding the mechanisms underpinning iron supplementation at different hemoglobin levels would help inform how far findings can be extrapolated.

8.4 SUMMARY

In this chapter, we discussed several additional designs, including traditional designs for individual data (case studies, case-crossover study), hybrid designs (pragmatic trials, doubly randomized preference trials, systematic reviews, meta-analysis), and quasi-experimental designs. It is worth disclaiming that this taxonomy is imperfect: many other epidemiologists would not classify meta-analysis as a hybrid design, as we have here, for example. And others do not consider quasi-experimental studies to be "designs" at all but rather analytic approaches to observational data.

REFERENCES

Bärnighausen, T., Oldenburg, C., Tugwell, P., Bommer, C., Ebert, C., Barreto, M., . . . Vollmer, S. (2017). Quasi-experimental study designs series-paper 7: Assessing the assumptions. *Journal of Clinical Epidemiology*, *89*, 53–66. doi:10.1016/j.jclinepi.2017.02.017

Bor, J. (2016). Capitalizing on natural experiments to improve our understanding of population health. *American Journal of Public Health*, *106*(8), 1388–1389. doi:10.2105/AJPH.2016.303294

Bynum, W. (2013). In retrospect: On the mode of communication of cholera. *Nature*, *495*, 169–170.

Centers for Disease Control (CDC). (1981). Pneumocystis pneumonia—Los Angeles. *MMWR Morbidity and Mortality Weekly Report*, *30*(21), 250–252.

Deer, B. (2011). How the case against the MMR vaccine was fixed. *British Medical Journal*, *342*, c5347. doi:10.1136/bmj.c5347

Godlee, F., Smith, J., & Marcovitch, H. (2011). Wakefield's article linking MMR vaccine and autism was fraudulent. *British Medical Journal*, *342*, c7452. doi:10.1136/bmj. c7452

Grant, M. J., & Booth, A. (2009). A typology of reviews: An analysis of 14 review types and associated methodologies. *Health Information Library Journal*, *26*(2), 91–108. doi:10.1111/j.1471-1842.2009.00848.x

Greenland, S. (1994). Invited commentary: A critical look at some popular meta-analytic methods. *American Journal of Epidemiology*, *140*(3), 290–296.

Hernán, M. A., & Robins, J. M. (2006). Instruments for causal inference: An epidemiologist's dream? *Epidemiology*, *17*(4), 360–372.

Johnson, S. B. (2006). *The ghost map: The story of London's most terrifying epidemic—and how it changed science, cities and the modern world*. New York: Riverhead.

Maclure, M. (1991). The case-crossover design: A method for studying transient effects on the risk of acute events. *American Journal of Epidemiology*, *133*(2), 144–153.

Maclure, M. (2007). "Why me?" versus "why now?"—differences between operational hypotheses in case-control versus case-crossover studies. *Pharmacoepidemiology and Drug Safety*, *16*(8), 850–853. doi:10.1002/pds.1438

Maclure, M., & Mittleman, M. A. (2000). Should we use a case-crossover design? *Annual Review of Public Health*, *21*, 193–221. doi:10.1146/annurev.publhealth.21.1.193

Mittleman, M. A., Maclure, M., Tofler, G. H., Sherwood, J. B., Goldberg, R. J., & Muller, J. E. (1993). Triggering of acute myocardial infarction by heavy physical exertion. Protection against triggering by regular exertion. Determinants of Myocardial Infarction Onset Study Investigators. *New England Journal of Medicine*, *329*(23), 1677–1683. doi:10.1056/NEJM199312023292301

Moher, D., Liberati, A., Tetzlaff, J., Altman, D. G., & Group, P. (2009). Preferred reporting items for systematic reviews and meta-analyses: The PRISMA statement. *Annals of Internal Medicine, 151*(4), 264–269, W264.

Nissen, T., & Wynn, R. (2014). The history of the case report: A selective review. *JRSM Open, 5*(4), 2054270414523410. doi:10.1177/2054270414523410

Ramsay, M. A. (2006). John Snow, MD: Anaesthetist to the Queen of England and pioneer epidemiologist. *Proceedings of the Baylor University Medical Center, 19*(1), 24–28.

Reeves, S., Koppel, I., Barr, H., Freeth, D., & Hammick, M. (2002). Twelve tips for undertaking a systematic review. *Medical Teacher, 24*(4), 358–363. doi:10.1080/01421590220145707

Rothman, K. J., Greenland, S., & Lash, T. L. (2008). *Modern epidemiology* (3rd ed.). Philadelphia: Lippincott Williams & Wilkins.

Scott, I., Greenberg, P., Poole, P., & Campbell, D. (2006). Cautionary tales in the interpretation of systematic reviews of therapy trials. *Internal Medicine Journal, 36*(9), 587–599. doi:10.1111/j.1445-5994.2006.01140.x

Snow, J. (1855). *On the mode of communication of cholera.* (2nd ed.) (pp. 74–75). London.

From Patients to Policy

Causal Impact

From Exposures to Interventions

In this chapter, we briefly discuss the *Causal Impact approach* to epidemiologic research. The Causal Impact framework outlines how we can move from internally valid estimates to externally valid estimates and, even further, to valid estimates of the effects of population interventions (Westreich et al., 2016). Broadly, such work—done within the Causal Impact framework or in some other way—is essential if we want the results of our experimental or observational studies to directly inform public health policy decisions. Thus, the bulk of this chapter can be seen as outlining an approach to epidemiologic methods relevant to implementation science.

9.1 THE CAUSAL IMPACT FRAMEWORK

Consider a randomized trial of pre-exposure prophylaxis (PrEP) for HIV compared to placebo: PrEP is (at the time of this writing) use of a daily anti-retroviral pill to reduce the chances that an exposure to HIV (as the result of unprotected sexual intercourse, for example) will result in an infection. Suppose the results of this trial show a strong protective effect of PrEP on the risk of HIV acquisition among trial participants, compared to placebo. Suppose further that the trial had no missing data and no measurement error, and in general can be assumed internally valid.

Before these trial results can be considered a sufficient evidence base to support the implementation of PrEP interventions, we must assess how such results might apply to a real-world setting—say, all people at risk of HIV infection in the entire United States. We consider this issue in two steps. First, we'll consider how well the results from the trial population approximate results in a given target population (external validity). Second, we'll consider how the effects of scale-up of PrEP in the real world might diverge from the results seen in the trial (population intervention impact). These considerations, while critical in bridging from trial evidence (or evidence from a well-conducted observational study) to policy, are frequently overlooked by epidemiologists. This may be because the methods used to assess them are not part of the traditional epidemiologic toolbox.

Epidemiology by Design: A Causal Approach to the Health Sciences. Daniel Westreich, Oxford University Press (2020). © Oxford University Press.
DOI: 10.1093/oso/9780190665760.001.0001

9.1.1 External Validity

The majority of work on causal inference focuses on internal validity: the validity of a causal effect estimate in the study sample (i.e., the data under study). However, no causal effect is fully specified unless we define a target population for that causal effect (Maldonado & Greenland, 2002). By target population we here mean specifically the population in whom we ultimately want causal knowledge—not necessarily just those who we are studying, but a larger group of people who may not be represented perfectly by the study sample (Westreich, Edwards, Lesko, Cole, & Stuart, 2019). For example, if the study sample for our hypothetical study included 2,000 Americans at risk of HIV, but we were studying these individuals to make decisions about all Americans at risk of HIV, then we could consider that latter group ("all Americans at risk of HIV") to be our target population. Unless the population enrolled in the randomized trial is identical to or representative of the target population (and, as we will argue later, neither case is likely), then the effect observed in the study sample may not apply in the target population.

Consider a simple example of how an effect in a study sample might not apply to a target population. Suppose that our study sample (again, the trial participants) has more older participants than younger participants compared to the target population of interest. This might happen if older people were more likely to consent to participate in the trial. Then suppose that, in subgroup analysis of this trial, we find that the effect of PrEP is much stronger in younger people compared to older people, that is there is effect measure modification (EMM) by age. If both these things are true, then there is EMM (or subgroup effects) on the scale of interest by some factor Z, and the effect in each subgroup (younger, older) can be assumed to be correct for the study sample. But also, the distribution of Z is different in the study sample and target population and so we should not expect the overall effect measured in the trial to be the same as we would have observed had, counter to fact, the trial been conducted in the target population.

9.1.2 Population Intervention Impact

Typically, the effect estimated in a randomized trial or observation study is a sample average causal effect. For our trial, that would be the comparison between "What is the risk of HIV infection if everyone in the trial sample was assigned to use PrEP?" and "What is the risk of HIV infection if everyone was assigned to use placebo?" However, public health policy to promote PrEP will not promote a placebo as an alternative; moreover, PrEP may not be recommended universally by clinicians to their patients and (among those patients to whom PrEP is recommended) may be taken up at different rates than seen in the trial. Finally, patterns of adherence to PrEP as well as the ability to counsel individuals to be more adherent may well differ between an experimental (possibly academic) setting and a scaled-up, universal access setting delivered by a different group of people.

Here enters a consideration of *population intervention estimate* (Hubbard & Laan, 2008), in which we consider the causal effect of an intervention applied to a specific population with a given distribution of an exposure we want to intervene against. The differences in assumptions between the effects of possible population interventions and more traditional estimates of the effects of exposures is often sharper in observational settings. For example, consider the sample average causal effect (i.e., the average causal effect described in Chapter 3, estimated in the study sample) typically estimated in an observational study of the impact of smoking on 5-year risk of death. That sample average causal effect is (generally) a comparison between "What is the 5-year risk of death if everyone was a smoker at baseline?" and "What is the 5-year risk of death if everyone was a nonsmoker at baseline?" (or "if everyone quit smoking at baseline?").

Such a sample average causal effect considers the impact of the exposure of smoking. But suppose we want to study the population impact of widespread smoking cessation interventions in the study population. Then our causal effect might compare "What is the 5-year risk of death we would expect in the observed population, given the observed levels of smoking?" with "What is the 5-year risk of death we would expect in the observed population, under the levels of smoking we would see if we offered individualized smoking cessation counseling and support to all smokers in that population?" Later, we explore the differences between the first comparison (the effects of an exposure) and the latter (the effects of an intervention) in greater detail: here we want you to see that the two comparisons ask quite different questions.

9.1.3 Causal Impact

Because of both questionable external validity and unrealistic interventions in the trial setting, the real-world population impact of a PrEP intervention is extremely unlikely to be identical to what is seen in a typical trial setting in which we randomized PrEP against placebo, 1:1. While the comparison of "all those who agreed to be in the trial assigned to PrEP, under experimental conditions" with "all those who agreed to be in the trial assigned to placebo, under experimental conditions" may be a good starting point for making policy, we should not naïvely assume that an estimate from such a traditional study is the only thing we need to start making decisions (e.g., when choosing between several possible interventions or as input to cost-effectiveness models).

We should emphasize that randomized trials can ask questions which are more directly relevant to policy than the hypothetical trial we have just outlined. Randomized trials can test many treatment plans, including dynamic treatment plans that alter treatments based on exposure values. Likewise, pragmatic trials can explore scaled-up interventions in highly unselected populations (Ford & Norrie, 2016; Thorpe et al., 2009): trials for HIV prevention in sub-Saharan Africa can enroll hundreds of thousands of people. We do not mean to discount such approaches. However, here we concentrate on classic, individually randomized clinical trials for two reasons: first, because they are far more widespread than alternatives and are still widely considered a gold standard of evidence. And second, because understanding why such trials may not produce policy-ready evidence is a good way to deepen our understanding of the advantages of more innovative study designs.

In the remainder of this chapter, we will expand briefly on both the issue of external validity and population intervention impact.

9.2 EXTERNAL VALIDITY

The majority of work on causal inference—and most of this book—focuses on internal validity: the validity of a causal effect estimate in the data under study (the study sample). But it remains notable that many epidemiologic studies that purport to estimate causal effects do not specifically call out the target population of interest, leaving the target population implied—often in ways that are questionable.

9.2.1 What Is the Target Population?

As noted earlier, the target population is the population that the researcher wants to understand better and apply the study results to, through examination of the study sample. Sometimes the study sample—for example, the participants in the randomized trial—is exactly equal to the target population, but this is not typical for several reasons. First, randomized trials tend to (though do not always) overenroll certain demographic groups: including younger people more than older people, healthy people more than sick people, and men more than women (Lee, Alexander, Hammill, Pasquali, & Peterson, 2001; Menezes et al., 2011; Susukida, Crum, Ebnesajjad, Stuart, & Mojtabai, 2017). In addition, any randomized trial which requires individual informed consent will almost certainly not include everyone approached to participate in the trial.

Rather than argue that the target population is exactly equal to the study sample, investigators sometimes argue that the study sample is representative of the target population, which would be true if, for instance, the study population were randomly sampled from the target population. Similarly, this is unlikely to be true, both because specific types of people tend to participate in trials (e.g., people with "health-seeking" behavior patterns) and, additionally, because trials sometimes deliberately recruit people at high risk of the outcome under study to enhance statistical power.

Thus, the target population may differ substantially from the study: the two may well have different distributions of covariates. If those covariates are EMMs (Chapters 5 and 6) for the causal effect being estimated in the study sample, then the effect estimated in the study sample may not represent the effect we would have seen if the same study had, counter-to-fact, been performed in the target population. Conducting trials in highly representative samples may sidestep

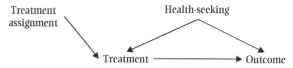

Figure 9.1 A directed acyclic graph for a randomized trial.

this problem for the intended target population but not for other possible target populations.

9.2.2 Varieties of External Validity

There are two types of external validity: generalizability and transportability. *Generalizability* is the case in which a study sample is entirely contained within the target population. For example, we wish to learn about individuals in Kenya (our target population), and so we conduct a trial among Kenyan volunteers (our study sample): since all Kenyan volunteers are individuals in Kenya, this is a case of generalizability. *Transportability* is any other case: that is, any case in which the study sample is *not* entirely contained within the target population. For example, we wish to know whether our Kenyan trial is valid in Uganda or if our observational study in North Carolina applies to South Carolina.

There are more similarities than differences between generalizability and transportability; that said, generalizability is conceptually easier. For this reason we will focus chiefly on generalizability for the remainder of this section.

9.2.3 Causal Approaches to Generalizability

The first thing that is worth observing about generalizability is that it can be thought of as a problem of missing data and expressed straightforwardly in a causal directed acyclic graph (DAG). We show two versions of a DAG for a randomized trial in Figures 9.1 and 9.2. Figure 9.1 shows the treatment assignment process, which affects true treatment status; the *true* treatment status with an arrow into the outcome; and the possible confounders of the true treatment–outcome relationship, such as a tendency toward health-seeking behavior. In Figure 9.2, we show a simplified version of the same DAG: dropping the arrow from Treatment assignment to Treatment is valid under perfect compliance with assigned treatment regimen, which we assume hereafter.

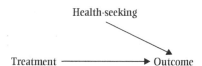

Figure 9.2 A directed acyclic graph for a randomized trial under simplifying assumptions (see text).

Note that in Figure 9.2, we have drawn a DAG for the study sample: the fact of the restriction to only those who chose to be in the trial is not represented in the DAG. Suppose we are estimating a causal effect for a target population that is a superset of the study sample—for example, if the study sample is residents of North Carolina and the target population is the entire United States. In this case our DAG does not represent the causal effect of interest. Instead, consider a DAG for the target population which includes a node for sampling into the study, as in Figure 9.3, where we put a box around "In the trial ($S = 1$)" to indicate that we have (by necessity) restricted analysis to those who were sampled into the trial. This is equivalent to supposing that all exposure and outcome data on members of the target population except those in the study sample are missing (or, alternatively, not selected).

Figure 9.3 is a DAG that captures the notion of generalizability in a way nearly identical to selection bias or complete case analysis of missing data (Lesko et al., 2017; Pearl, 2015). Recall that, when assessing confounding, we want to ensure that there are no open backdoor paths between the treatment (or exposure) and the outcome (Greenland, Pearl, & Robins, 1999; Pearl, 1995). When assessing generalizability (or similarly, missing data), we need to ensure a different but parallel condition: no open backdoor paths between sampling (the $S = 1$ box) and the outcome (Lesko et al., 2017). Examination of Figure 9.3 shows that there is such a path through Health-seeking behavior; that path is [In the trial ($S = 1$)]←Health-seeking→Outcome.

Just as we need exchangeability between the two exposure groups for internal validity, we need exchangeability between the study sample and the target population (really, the study sample and the missing members of the target population) for external validity. And just as "no uncontrolled confounding" is a reasonable (though somewhat informal and possibly incomplete) way of thinking about the more formal construct of exchangeability, we might think of exchangeability for generalizability as "no uncontrolled effect measure modification" or "no differences in distributions of effect measure modifiers between the study sample and target population." However, this more informal condition may lead us astray in certain cases, and the DAG-based criterion may be preferable.

Thinking through other issues in internal validity can illuminate external validity as well. For example, if a study sample included no women over the age of 60, and the target population is 15% women over age 60, then we have an

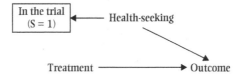

Figure 9.3 A directed acyclic graph for a randomized trial drawn in the target population, including a node for sampling into trial.

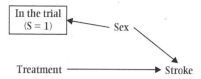

Figure 9.4 A directed acyclic graph for a randomized trial in which Sex affects entry to study sample.

issue of external positivity. As with internal positivity, we can address this issue through model extrapolation. Other identification conditions for internal validity, including consistency and no interference, have parallels for external validity (Hernán & Vanderweele, 2011; Lesko et al., 2017).

Finally, in the same way that randomization of treatment helps us meet numerous identification conditions in a single study, we can randomize our way to an expectation of external validity as well. If the study sample is indeed a simple random sample of the target population, then we should have exchangeability (in expectation) between individuals in the study sample and individuals in the target population, and we may meet additional identification conditions as well (target positivity, for example). Thus, we may wish to reconsider the idea that the randomized trial is the "gold standard" for inference: with respect to a specific target population, the gold standard for inference may well be a doubly randomized trial: random selection from the target population and random treatment assignment.

9.2.4 Quantitative Generalizability

A full and formal treatment of quantitative methods for generalizability (or transportability) of trial results to a target population is beyond the scope of this book. Briefly, however, existing methods make use of standardization. We addressed standardization in Chapter 6 as a way of addressing confounding in an observational study and remind you that standardization can be thought of as a kind of weighted averaging.

Here we give a simple example. Suppose we conduct our 5-year-long randomized trial (outcome: stroke), and, in the process of enrolling subjects from the general population, we oversample men such that the study sample is 75% men and 25% women, reflecting that randomized trials frequently—though by no means always—fail to include women commensurate with women's representation in the total population. Such a study—assuming perfect compliance with treatment assignment, as in Figure 9.2—might look like Figure 9.4. Data consistent with Figure 9.4 are shown in Table 9.1: sex affects stroke in that untreated men have a higher risk of stroke than untreated women. The fact that treatment affects stroke is shown in that risk differences for treatment are non-null. In addition, note that probability of treatment is 50% in both men and women: because of randomization, sex and treatment are unconditionally independent (i.e.,

Table 9.1 Data consistent with Figure 9.4

Men	Stroke	No stroke	Total	Risk	RD
Treated	75	1,425	1,500	5%	−15%
Untreated	300	1,200	1,500	20%	

Women	Stroke	No stroke	Total	Risk	RD
Treated	25	475	500	5%	−5%
Untreated	50	450	500	10%	

All	Stroke	No stroke	Total	Risk	RD
Treated	100	1,900	2,000	5%	−12.5%
Untreated	350	1,650	2,000	17.5%	

unassociated), shown in the DAG by the lack of an arrow from Sex to Treatment (and no backdoor paths between them, either).

From data in Table 9.1, we calculate the 5-year risk difference in men is −15%, in women is −5%, and overall is −12.5%. Because this is a trial and there is no confounding present in these data, we can either take the data combined across Men and Women (shown as "All," in Table 9.1), or alternatively take a weighted average of the risk differences, specifically −15% * 3,000/4,000 + −5% * 1,000/4,000. However, in the presence of confounding, neither approach would be guaranteed to work, and more typical standardization approaches must be used.

Now suppose our target population is 50% men and 50% women: What overall effect would we expect to see in that target population? The easiest thing to do is to simply make a new table (of arbitrary size n) that depicts the distribution of sex in the target population (again, 50% men, 50% women). Ideally, of course, we would generate this new table by taking a random sample of the target population, but we can also just create a table that reflects our knowledge that the target population has equal numbers of men and women. The corresponding DAG would not have an arrow from Sex to selection into the trial, as shown in Figure 9.5. One easy way to create such a table is to copy Table 9.1, but simply increase number of women such that there are the same number of treated and untreated men and women. In this case, we can simply upweight all the women by 3, as shown in Table 9.2. To determine whether these new women should be in the "stroke" or "no stroke" column, we rely on the subgroup-specific risk estimates we calculated in the trial.

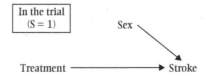

Figure 9.5 A randomized trial in which differential sampling due to Sex has been corrected.

Table 9.2 DATA CONSISTENT WITH FIGURE 9.5

Men	Stroke	No stroke	Total	Risk	RD
Treated	75	1,425	1,500	5%	−15%
Untreated	300	1,200	1,500	20%	

Women	Stroke	No stroke	Total	Risk	RD
Treated	75	1,425	1,500	5%	−5%
Untreated	150	1,350	1,500	10%	

All	Stroke	No stroke	Total	Risk	RD
Treated	150	2,850	3,000	5%	−10%
Untreated	450	2,550	3,000	15%	

Now that we have equal numbers of men and women in our hypothetical target population, we can simply combine them and assess the overall effect again: which yields a risk difference of −10%, instead of the previous value of −12.5%. (Again, and alternatively, we could have calculated this target risk difference as −15% * 3,000/6,000 + −5% * 3,000/6,000. And again, both these very simple methods only work in the absence of confounding.)

Is this a meaningful difference? It might be: it moves the number needed to treat from $(1/0.125 =)$ 8 to $(1/0.100 =)$ 10, which could easily impact overall cost-effectiveness of the intervention. But regardless, the principle remains useful: when the distribution of an effect measure modifier changes from the study sample to the target population, we should expect the effect estimate to change as well. We leave it to you to estimate the overall effect in a population comprising 25% men and 75% women.

We have shown that when distribution of an EMM is different in the study sample and target population, we should expect to see different effect estimates in each. Is such a situation common? Recall from Chapter 6 that when (i) a causal effect is non-null and (ii) the risk in the unexposed changes, we will see differences in causal effects in either the risk difference or risk ratio (or both)— that is, EMM on at least one scale. Now consider further that, as often as not, randomized trials oversample individuals at high risk of the outcome in order to enhance study power and efficiency: HIV vaccine trials, for example, often only enroll individuals who admit to risky sexual practices that may put them at higher risk of HIV acquisition. Finally, recall our earlier argument that the study sample is only rarely the same as the trial population. Thus, for many trials, the true effect of an intervention in the (usually unnamed) target population will differ at least somewhat from what is estimated in the study itself.

Again, a more sophisticated treatment of the generalization and/or transport of the results of randomized or observational trials is beyond our scope; however, there are approaches using inverse probability weights (Cole & Stuart, 2010; Westreich, Edwards, Lesko, Stuart, & Cole, 2017) as well as other methods in a rapidly expanding literature.

9.2.5 Summary

There is a growing epidemiologic literature on external validity, much of it too new to be included in this work. One critical takeaway for readers is that it is important to specify an intended target population when publishing the results of a randomized trial or observational study. Another is that external validity is *specific to the target population being considered*: too often, usage of "external validity" and "generalizability" in the epidemiologic literature omit a description of the specific target population of interest. Since external validity of a specific study can vary enormously from one target population to another, readers should interrogate the idea that we can judge study results as being "externally valid" in some absolute or abstract sense (Westreich et al., 2019). Finally, while we have focused on external validity of randomized trials, similar considerations apply to observational studies.

9.3 POPULATION INTERVENTION EFFECTS

If we understand what the results of a randomized trial or observational study might mean in terms of public health policy, the necessary first caution is that the results of a single trial are rarely, if ever, the basis on which to make policy. Then we must consider the external validity of our results, as we discussed earlier. Subsequently, we must consider the distance between the effect estimated in a randomized trial or observational study and the effect which would be observed under a public health policy.

There are numerous reasons why such an effect estimate may not translate directly to real-world conditions. Consider a simple intervention—say, a vaccine, albeit one that requires two doses to take full effect—that has been found to have a strong protective effect in a randomized trial and then was transported to a target population of interest (e.g., using inverse probability of sampling weights; Cole & Stuart, 2010). The effect being estimated in the target population is therefore a contrast between "What if everyone was assigned to receive the vaccine?" compared with "What if everyone was assigned to receive the placebo?" Why might this effect differ from the effect of a public health policy that might follow—for example, the policy, "give this vaccine to everyone in the target population"? Some reasons might include:

1. The target population is not receiving a placebo currently. If the placebo had any effect on the risk of the outcome—for example, people who received the placebo had slightly lower risk than they would have if, counter to fact, they had received nothing at all—then the effect under the policy will differ from the trial effect.
2. It is likely that nearly everyone in the trial received at least the first dose of the vaccine or placebo because in such a trial the first vaccine dose would be given within minutes of randomization. In a scale-up, it is

extremely likely that some people who should receive the vaccine never receive even their first dose.

3. Among those who receive their first dose, the conditions of a trial (such as aggressive and frequent follow-up of research subjects) might make some participants more likely to return for the second dose. In a scale-up, those trial conditions will not hold, which could reduce the probability that people return for their second dose. Such an effect might be even sharper in a trial of a drug which must be taken daily, in which adherence must be maintained actively over time. On the other hand, if a trial is completed and the outcome was positive, that messaging might increase the number of people who return for a second shot. (After all, "this works!" is a more compelling message than "we're not sure if this vaccine is any better than salt water!")

While the first point (placebo-control) is unlikely to apply in an observational context, the other two points may be equally relevant in an observational setting, which will present additional problems as well.

9.3.1 Exposures and Population Interventions

As we noted earlier, very often people estimating a causal effect of an exposure in an observational setting will estimate a sample average causal effect, which compares risks in the study sample (or target population) if everyone was exposed versus if no one was exposed. For example, an observational study in which the main exposure was incident pregnancy would ask about risk if everyone in the study had experienced a new pregnancy compared to if no one in the study had experienced an incident pregnancy. While such effects are typically not exactly what would be observed under trial conditions in that they are conditional on covariates, they are, broadly, a similar contrast to the sample average causal effects sometimes estimated in trials.

To illustrate this comparison, we introduce Figure 9.6 (adapted from Westreich, 2017): in panel a, we show the observed population (the circle) in which some minority of individuals are exposed (shaded section of circle) and the remainder are unexposed. A sample (or population) average causal effect, then, estimates Figure 9.6b, comparing the situation in which everyone is exposed (left, fully shaded circle) to that in which everyone is unexposed (or exposed to some alternative; right, unshaded circle). In all circles the risk of the outcome is not shown; rather, the circles just represent the contrast of exposure distributions.

What is striking about these comparisons is that both sides of each are "counterfactual" in the literal sense of being *counter-to-fact*. In truth (panel a of Figure 9.6), not everyone in the observational cohort experienced exposure; nor did everyone experience nonexposure. To be more specific, suppose we are estimating the effect of initiating smoking at least a pack of cigarettes a day on risk of 20-year all-cause mortality drawn from a population in which—say—20% of people start smoking at this level in the year before baseline. In such a case, we might well estimate an average causal effect of smoking: that is, the 20-year mortality risk had everyone started smoking, compared with the 20-year mortality risk had no one started smoking. Already the contradiction is evident: in reality, only 20% of people started smoking, and yet we are asking a question comparing two things which did not happen (all started smoking, and no one started).

How are we to interpret such a causal effect? While this is not strictly interpretable as an individual causal effect (Chapter 3), treating this average causal effect as a first guess at the individual causal effect is at least reasonable and consistent with the way such a finding is used: to inform clinical and individual decision making about the danger (or benefit) of an exposure (or treatment). For this reason, we call such causal effects *exposure effects*. Exposure effects will be most useful when a patient resembles those in your study (or you have generalized your study results to a population that looks like the patient)—although again, we cannot identify the causal effects in an individual.

Now instead consider a decision maker trying to decide how much of a public health problem is represented by initiation of smoking in this population and which resources to devote to eliminating smoking. How does this average causal effect inform her decision making? Policy makers must operate starting with the world as it is: Figure 9.6a. Yet again, neither side of the comparison in Figure 9.6b is observed (in particular, neither looks like Figure 9.6a).

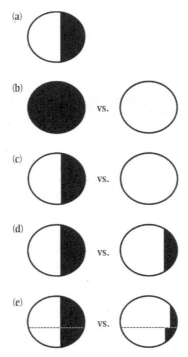

Figure 9.6 Exposure and population intervention effects.

Are there causal effects that might be more useful to their work? Population intervention effects are one alternative: in general, they compare the observed exposure distribution in the real (observed) population with some alternative (Hubbard & van der Laan, 2008). We have already introduced one such measure: the population attributable fraction (Chapter 3), which compares the risk under the observed exposure distribution to the risk in the same population if no one was exposed. Using our circle diagrams, this comparison looks like Figure 9.6c. The population attributable fraction, it should be noted, is just one way of conceptualizing this comparison; we could also calculate a risk difference or ratio between the two circles. Thus we call this class of comparisons *population attributable effects*. We also note that because we are thinking broadly about potential interventions, we would prefer risk difference measures here (see Chapters 2 and 3).

The population attributable effect can—broadly—be thought of as the impact of the best possible intervention, one which removes the exposure entirely (without side effects). Of course, it is unrealistic to imagine removing the exposure entirely in many situations. Consider current smokers: typically fewer than 100% of current smokers even wish to quit smoking; among those who do, our best smoking cessation interventions are no more than perhaps 25% effective. This leads us to a second population intervention effect, shown in Figure 9.6d: the *generalized intervention effect*, which compares total population risk under the observed exposure distribution to a counterfactual in which some (where "all" is a special case of "some") exposure has been removed from the population—at random from among exposed individuals. Generalized intervention effects will be increasingly interpretable in real-world (or policy) terms as the percentage of the exposure removed can be directly related to a specific, realistic, and empirically tested real-world intervention: as with the immediately preceding example, because we have few (if any) smoking cessation interventions which are 50% effective but more which are 25% effective, a generalized intervention effect looking at a 25% reduction in smoking is likely more useful to policy makers than one looking at a 50% reduction.

More realistic still is that interventions rarely work equally well on all members of the population and may in fact have dramatically different effects depending on well-measured characteristics of individuals, such as self-reported sex or age. The *dynamic intervention effect* (Figure 9.6e) allows an intervention to remove exposure differentially by individual participant characteristics and can be used to model targeted interventions.

Here, we wish to briefly observe that there are significant implications of this model of thinking for the number needed to treat (NNT; see Chapter 2). An NNT calculated from an observational study is typically calculated using the sample average causal effect from that study—that is, it is calculated from an estimated effect of an exposure. But the effect of an exposure is not necessarily the same as the effect of a treatment for (or intervention against) that exposure: as we have just observed, treatments are rarely 100% effective. Thus, for any real treatment, the NNT derived from a comparison in which one side is "no exposure remains" seems likely to be overly optimistic.

As well, different treatments are applied to different populations. While a to-bacco education program is applied to the general population, tobacco cessation activities are applied only to current smokers. Thus, uses of NNT which do not specify the details of the treatment or population being treated are difficult to interpret.

Finally, we would be remiss not to add that anyone interested in intervening to improve population health would be well served to read (or reread!) Geoffrey Rose's towering and influential paper, "Sick Individuals and Sick Populations," published in the *International Journal of Epidemiology* in 1985.

9.4 THE HIERARCHY OF STUDY DESIGNS

A web image search for "hierarchy of the study designs" or "hierarchy of evidence" will yield a range of figures with some commonalities and some differences. Most of those hierarchies of study designs will place meta-analysis (often meta-analysis of randomized trials, only) at the top, followed by randomized trials, prospective observational cohort studies, and case-control studies, then followed in some order by case series and reports, editorials, expert opinions, and animal or in vitro studies.

While there are some exceptions, many of these hierarchies do not specify what sorts of questions they are addressing with their study designs, although often the estimation of causal effects is implied. Nor do such hierarchies typically acknowledge what metrics they are using to judge which study designs are better, though often—equally implied—the answer is internal validity alone. We offer several counterpoints.

First, different study designs are best for different questions. If your scientific question is "Can a particular disease X ever present with symptom Y? And therefore should disease X be in the differential diagnosis for patients with symptom Y?" then likewise a report of several cases can answer the question. A randomized trial to answer the question would be unethical if not impossible—but it is also unnecessary: case reports were perfectly valid for addressing the question at hand. On the other hand, if you want to know the effect on cancer survival of a new chemotherapy option compared to standard of care, then a randomized trial or prospective observational cohort study may be a better option.

Second, for comparative studies of causality—treatment versus placebo or nontreatment, exposed versus unexposed—the *unexamined presumption* that a randomized trial belongs above prospective observational cohort studies represents a failure to consider metrics beyond internal validity. It is straightforward to construct a situation in which the validity of an observational study is equal to that of a randomized trial *for a particular target population*, despite uncontrolled confounding in the observational study. This might be the case if, for example, the randomized trial was conducted in a highly skewed sample of the target population while the observational study was conducted in a representative sample of the target. When we consider not just internal validity, but total validity with respect to a specific target population, the presumed preference for a randomized trial may start to weaken.

As discussed earlier, pragmatic randomized trials—conducted in less-selected populations than typical randomized clinical trials and using interventions that closely mirror a scaled-up intervention—may represent a middle-way between internally and externally valid results with immediate relevance to implementation. Some quasi-experimental designs may have similar properties.

9.5 SUMMARY

In recent years, epidemiology has often focused only on issues of estimating internally valid effects of exposures. But epidemiology—and public health—can produce evidence more relevant to public health policy change by considering not just internal validity, but also external validity (i.e., how the results in the study apply in other populations) and population intervention effects (i.e., the impact of realistic interventions against the exposures of interest).

REFERENCES

Cole, S. R., & Stuart, E. A. (2010). Generalizing evidence from randomized clinical trials to target populations: The ACTG 320 trial. *American Journal of Epidemiology, 172*(1), 107–115. doi:10.1093/aje/kwq084

Ford, I., & Norrie, J. (2016). Pragmatic trials. *New England Journal of Medicine, 375*(5), 454–463. doi:10.1056/NEJMra1510059

Greenland, S., Pearl, J., & Robins, J. M. (1999). Causal diagrams for epidemiologic research. *Epidemiology, 10*(1), 37–48.

Hernán, M. A., & Vanderweele, T. J. (2011). Compound treatments and transportability of causal inference. *Epidemiology, 22*(3), 368–377. doi:10.1097/EDE.0b013e3182109296

Hubbard, A. E., & van der Laan, M. J. (2008). Population intervention models in causal inference. *Biometrika, 95*(1), 35–47.

Lee, P. Y., Alexander, K. P., Hammill, B. G., Pasquali, S. K., & Peterson, E. D. (2001). Representation of elderly persons and women in published randomized trials of acute coronary syndromes. *Journal of the American Medical Association, 286*(6), 708–713.

Lesko, C. R., Buchanan, A. L., Westreich, D., Edwards, J. K., Hudgens, M. G., & Cole, S. R. (2017). Generalizing study results: A potential outcomes perspective. *Epidemiology, 28*(4), 553–561. doi:10.1097/EDE.0000000000000664

Maldonado, G., & Greenland, S. (2002). Estimating causal effects. *International Journal of Epidemiology, 31*(2), 422–429.

Menezes, P., Eron, J. J., Jr., Leone, P. A., Adimora, A. A., Wohl, D. A., & Miller, W. C. (2011). Recruitment of HIV/AIDS treatment-naive patients to clinical trials in the highly active antiretroviral therapy era: Influence of gender, sexual orientation and race. *HIV Medicine, 12*(3), 183–191. doi:10.1111/j.1468-1293.2010.00867.x

Pearl, J. (1995). Causal diagrams for empirical research. *Biometrika, 82*(4), 669–688.

Pearl, J. (2015). Generalizing experimental findings. *Journal of Causal Inference, 3*(2), 259–266.

Rose, G. (1985). Sick individuals and sick populations. *International Journal of Epidemiology*, *14*(1), 32–38.

Susukida, R., Crum, R. M., Ebnesajjad, C., Stuart, E. A., & Mojtabai, R. (2017). Generalizability of findings from randomized controlled trials: Application to the National Institute of Drug Abuse Clinical Trials Network. *Addiction*, *112*(7), 1210–1219. doi:10.1111/add.13789

Thorpe, K. E., Zwarenstein, M., Oxman, A. D., Treweek, S., Furberg, C. D., Altman, D. G., . . . Chalkidou, K. (2009). A pragmatic-explanatory continuum indicator summary (PRECIS): A tool to help trial designers. *Journal of Clinical Epidemiology*, *62*(5), 464–475. doi:10.1016/j.jclinepi.2008.12.011

Westreich, D. (2017). From patients to policy: Population intervention effects in epidemiology. *Epidemiology*, *28*(4), 525–528. doi:10.1097/EDE.0000000000000648

Westreich, D., Edwards, J. K., Lesko, C. R., Cole, S. R., & Stuart, E. A. (2019). Target validity and the hierarchy of study designs. *American Journal of Epidemiology*, *188*(2), 438–443. doi:10.1093/aje/kwy228

Westreich, D., Edwards, J. K., Lesko, C. R., Stuart, E., & Cole, S. R. (2017). Transportability of trial results using inverse odds of sampling weights. *American Journal of Epidemiology*, *186*(8), 1010–1014. doi:10.1093/aje/kwx164

Westreich, D., Edwards, J. K., Rogawski, E. T., Hudgens, M. G., Stuart, E. A., & Cole, S. R. (2016). Causal impact: Epidemiological approaches for a public health of consequence. *American Journal of Public Health*, *106*(6), 1011–1012. doi:10.2105/AJPH.2016.303226

INDEX

Note: Page numbers followed by *b*, *f*, and *t* indicate boxes, figures, and tables, respectively.

For the benefit of digital users, indexed terms that span two pages (e.g., 52–53) may, on occasion, appear on only one of those pages.